Low Carb

Ketogenic Diet to Overcome Belly Fat, Lose Pounds and Live Healthy

Brian Adams

© Copyright 2015 - All rights reserved.

Brian Adams

Readers acknowledge that the author is not engaging in the rendering of legal, financial, medical or professional advice.

By reading this document, the reader agrees that under no circumstances are we responsible for any losses, direct or indirect, which are incurred as a result of the use of information contained within this document, including, but not limited to, — errors, omissions, or inaccuracies.

Table of Contents

Introduction

Fat bodies and obesity are something that everybody loathes; but given today's hectic lifestyles and junk food dependence, they have become part of an inescapable scenario. Right from children to adults to old people, obesity is now grappling a wide array of people, with most of them complaining about belly fat and a lack of energy.

Continued obesity can have a negative impact on the body and cause people to develop secondary health conditions such as diabetes and cardiovascular illnesses. The need of the hour is to therefore come up with a diet solution, which will help people lose their belly fat, lose those extra pounds and attain good health.

One such diet is the Ketogenic diet, which is now gaining popularity owing to its high-level success rate. In this eBook, we look at the ketogenic diet in detail and cover it's meaning, its various aspects, and also its main purpose. We also have a look at some basic ketogenic recipes for you to give it a try.

Brian Adams

Chapter 1: Ketogenic Diet And Other Related FAQ's

In this first chapter, we will look at a few standard questions about the diet and answer them to help you understand the concept better.

What is the ketogenic diet?

The ketogenic diet refers to a high fat and low carbohydrate diet, which is meant to help the liver produce ketones. Ketones are responsible for causing the body to burn fat, as a means of supplying energy, as opposed to burning carbohydrates.

Our bodies burn carbohydrates and turn it into glucose, which is used up by the body to maintain a study supply of energy. But this glucose can get stored as fat and cause people to turn obese. The Ketogenic diet, on the other hand, helps the body in getting rid of the excess fat and also allows it to not store any new fat.

Why was it invented?

The ketogenic diet was invented, as a means to treat children with severe epilepsy. The diet promotes the release of ketones, which is responsible for lowering the risk of developing seizures. Ketones are nothing but a set of chemicals, which when released go to the brain and replace the glucose present there and all over the body.

This is only possible when the patient is administered a diet low in carbs and high in fat and so, it caught the fancy of dieticians and dieters, who thought of applying the concept to obese people, as they also needed their fat to be burned and not merely the carbohydrates.

When was it invented?

The diet is said to have been invented in the early 1920's and mainly for the sake of treating children with severe epilepsy. Although diet treatments were quite rare and people relied on medicines more, the ketogenic diet had shown a lot of potential and several tests were conducted on the same, which put forth several possibilities.

Ketones are said to be good for the body in more ways than one and are a much better alternative to glucose. Ever since, the diet has evolved quite a bit and now incorporates several changes and has been adopted by people, keen on losing excess body weight and maintaining an ideal one.

Is it effective in weight loss?

Yes. It is quite effective in weight loss as the diet promotes the burning of existing body fat and utilizes it to supply energy. That way, not only is the existing fat being burnt away but the brain is also being trained to burn fat and not carbs. Once these fats are burnt and there is no carbs being reintroduced to the body, there is no chance of it being stored as fat. So it is a weight loss diet that will have not just short term, but long-term effects on the body as well.

Does it have any other benefits?

Yes. The diet also helps in lowering blood sugar levels. It helps in controlling the amount of sugar that is released in the blood stream and also helps in controlling the amount that is utilized by the body by helping in the secretion of insulin.

So the diet is adopted by obese diabetics, as it can help them have a control over their diabetes and also lose weight at the same time, which is not possible with most of the other types of diets. The diet also promotes in the building of lean muscles, as there is good amounts of proteins that are encouraged to be consumed.

Is there evidence available for its claims?

Yes. There are several study results that claim the diet to work on obesity and help people lose weight. There are also hundreds of testimonials available on the Internet that has been put up by satisfied ketogenic dieters. They claim to have not just lost excess weight but also prevented it from coming back on.

However, there have been no official studies or research conducted on the topic and such research has only been limited to the ones conducted by pediatricians on children. No such major breakthrough research has yet been sanctioned or conducted and remains to be inconclusive.

What foods are allowed in the diet?

The diet allows high fat and low carb ingredients in the ratios 4:1. But that is for a classic ketogenic diet. The one meant for weight loss incorporate 2:1 or even 1:1. So people are made to consume meats, dairy products, fruits, vegetables and nuts that have a high fat content and low carbohydrate content.

Apart from these beverages such as water, tea and juices are allowed provided they are low in carbs and mostly green tea and fresh fruit juices are encouraged. Spices and artificial sweeteners are also a part of the diet. (A more detailed list is provided in chapter 2 of this eBook.)

Can anybody take it up?

Yes. The diet is mostly meant for obese and overweight people, who are looking for a permanent weight loss solution and something that will allow them to maintain an ideal body weight. It is for people who do not have the time to exercise and burn away the carbs, glucose and fat from their bodies.

So it is meant for obese children who need to study, obese women, who need to take care of families, obese men, who do not have time owing to a busy work schedule, obese old people etc. it does not really have an age restriction, but in some cases, it might be important to first check with the physician.

Are there side effects?

Yes. As is with most other weight loss diets, the ketogenic diet also has a few side effects. But these side effects are mostly temporary and not something that might threaten life. These include nausea, constipation, frequent urination and dizziness. But these will occur only if the diet is not followed properly. If you will understand why these will happen and take precautions to prevent them from happening, then you will be able to successfully steer clear of these.

More on this is mentioned in chapter 4 of the eBook.

Can vegetarians and vegans take it up?

Yes. Although the diet focuses on the consumption of non-vegetarian foods, it is possible to consume only vegetables, fruits, nuts, seeds and dairy and cut the dairy out if it is a vegan diet.

Brian Adams

Chapter 2: Basic Principles of The Diet

In the previous chapter, we looked at what the ketogenic diet is all about and some of its other aspects. In this chapter, we have an in depth look at the basics of the diet and its various advantages. I will also give you a comprehensive shopping list for the diet.

Low carbs

The main principle of the diet is to allow very little carbohydrates to be present in it. This means that foods that contain sugars and starches are not allowed and even if they are, then they should be in very less quantity.

By consuming a low carb diet, the dieter can keep cardiovascular diseases at bay. These can generally come about owing to the consumption of foods laden with bad fats and sugars and since these are kept out of the diet, it helps in promoting good health.

Another advantage is that, it helps in keeping diabetes away. By consuming low carb foods, the body does not get an opportunity to store glucose, which is nothing but sugar. Therefore, there will not be any excess sugar in the blood stream and no risk of developing diabetes.

High fat

The main reason why fat is introduced to the body is so that, it can help in fighting away the existing fat. This is made possible as the ketones that are released start to burn the fat in the body to help supply energy.

But this fat is not bad fat but good fat. Bad fat refers to triglycerides, which can cause the body to develop cholesterol. Cholesterol is bad for the heart and can counter the effects of the diet. This form of cholesterol forming fat is known as long chain triglyceride or LCT.

The fat that is encouraged is MCT or medium chain triglycerides. This is a special type of fat and is derived from oils such as coconut oil. These are good fats and will not cause the body to undertake fat.

Omega 3 fatty acids are also promoted, as there is a lot of consumption of fish and fish products. These further help with maintaining a healthy body. Ideally, a person on the ketogenic diet should get no more than 50 grams of carbohydrates per day.

Adequate protein

Protein is extremely important for the body, as it can help in building strong muscles. Many times, if the body does not have enough glucose to burn for strength, then it starts to burn the muscles and use it up for energy. This problem can also occur with the ketogenic diet, where after all the fat has been burnt, the body might start to draw from muscles. However, this situation is countered by the use of adequate proteins, which not only assist in building new muscles but help in strengthening existing ones.

Proteins also help in keeping a person feeling full for a long time. So, by consuming foods rich in proteins, people can feel full and sated for a long time and successfully put an end to hunger pangs.

Advantages of the diet

Weight loss
The main advantage of the diet is that it helps in weight loss. The diet helps in losing those extra pounds and can also be used to maintain an ideal body weight. Apart from weight loss, it helps in maintaining a slim figure and there will be no fat, which will cause a bulge.

Diseases
The ketogenic diet helps people in remaining healthy. It cuts down on the risk of developing various illnesses such as diabetes, heart disease, certain types of cancers, bone related illnesses, joint pains etc. The diet is therefore meant to be continued and should not be stopped as soon as weight loss is attained.

Productivity
Since the diet promotes ketone release, which goes to the brain and replaces the glucose, people's mental power tends to increase. As per several studies, people who follow the ketogenic diet for a while have elevated levels of productivity and claim to perform tasks faster and in an efficient manner. This is also relevant in terms of children, as they will have better brain function and be able to concentrate better on their studies.

Appearance

With the help of the diet, women can attain a beautiful body. Thanks to the consumption of omega 3 fatty acids and cutting out of sugars, skin, hair and teeth will benefit and women can attain clear skin, silky mane and shiny teeth. The consumption of dairy products will also contribute towards the same.

Ketogenic diet shopping list

Meats

- Chicken - whole or parts, skinned and trimmed to your liking
- Beef steaks and tips, trimmed to your liking
- Bacon, ham and sausage, trimmed to your liking
- Pork loin, chops or steaks, trimmed to your liking
- Pork or beef ribs
- Beef or pork roasts, good quality
- Ground beef, good quality and made from fatty cuts
- Ground turkey, good quality and made from fatty cuts

Deli meats

- Cold cuts such as turkey breast and pastrami, with no sugar added in
- Pepperoni sticks or slices, trimmed to your liking
- Salami and bologna, trimmed to your liking
- Prosciutto, trimmed to your liking

Sea food

- Fresh or frozen prawns, deveined
- Fresh or frozen fish, ideally tuna, cod and sardines
- Tuna in oil or tuna water

- Cod liver oil
- Fresh or canned salmon
- Fresh or frozen scallops
- Fresh Crab or crab sticks, with no sugars added in

Dairy Products
- Fresh organic Eggs, duck, chicken
- Heavy cream
- Sour cream
- Cream cheese
- Grass fed butter
- Hard cheeses such as cheddar and parmesan
- Soft cheeses such an muenster and farmer
- Greek yogurt full fat with no sugar added

Low carbohydrate vegetables
- Bell peppers of all colors
- Broccoli
- Cabbage
- Cucumbers
- Zucchini
- Cauliflower
- Lettuce
- Leafy green vegetables such as spinach, curry leaves, fenugreek leaves and kale
- Onions and garlic, fresh not pastes or powders
- Sprouts for salads
- Summer squash such as gourds

Nuts and Seeds
- Nuts such as almonds, hazelnuts, pecans, walnuts, cashew nuts, and macadamia nuts.
- Seeds such as sunflower, flax seeds, pumpkin and sesame (black and white) seeds

Low carbohydrate fruits
- Avocados:
- Strawberries, raspberries, oranges and other such fruits that is mostly sour and not too sweet as they can contain lots of carbohydrates. Always remember to mix a fruit with a fat substance to help with the diet.

Seasonings
- Pickles or relish of your choice with no sugar added in, ideally radish, tuna or fish pickles
- Mustard, without any sugar or honey
- Apple cider vinegar, balsamic vinegar
- Tobacco sauce, hot sauce, chili sauce
- Salsa without sugar
- Sugar free soya sauce
- Low carb, sugar free mayonnaise
- Ranch dressing without sugar
- Capers
- Horseradish
- Green and black Olives
- Lemon or lime juice, no sugar added

Baking Ingredients
- Whey protein powder of your choice, plain, vanilla and chocolate flavors

- Splenda or other artificial sweeteners of your choice
- Xylitol and other sugar alcohol sweeteners of your choice
- Herbs and spices, spice rubs, sugar free
- Pure vanilla, lemon or almond extracts, sugar free
- Broths of your choice, sugar free
- Cocoa powder which is unsweetened
- Gelatin
- Xanthan gum for thickening and binding
- Extra-virgin olive oil
- Peanut oil, olive oil and coconut oil for cooking
- Sesame oil and olive oil for salad dressings
- Almond flour or other nut flours that are fresh

Others

- Tuna, salmon, crab, shrimp, sardines, anchovies, all canned
- Sausages
- Tomato pastes, purees and sauces, sugar free
- Pasta sauces and condiments, sugar free
- Pizza sauces and spreads, sugar free
- Sauerkrauts, sugar free, ideally cabbage
- Green chilies, sun dried peppers, chipotle peppers, dried mushrooms, sun dried artichoke hearts, sun-dried tomatoes
- Fresh chicken, beef, fish and/ or vegetable stock
- Nut butters without sugar such as cashew butter, almond butter, peanut butter, whipped cream and cream cheese without sugar

Chapter 3: Warnings and Precautions

Now that we looked at some basic recipes for you to try out, we will now look at some warnings and precautions to bear in mind, when you take up the ketogenic diet.

Physician

It is best that you consult a qualified physician before you take up the diet, as he will be able to guide you better. You can do your own research and come up with a plan no doubt, but you must also have it checked by the physician, as it will be better to get it approved first. He might also warn you against any of the side effects and correct the diet by adding or subtracting some of the things in your diet. You must also make him/ her fully aware of any other conditions that you may have, as it will be important to note it and then come up with a diet plan.

Monitoring

There should be consistent monitoring of all your vital statistics during the course of the diet. The dietician or physician must check for the levels of nutrients present in your body and make sure that you are getting whatever is needed by you to maintain a healthy body. You must not miss any sessions, as it will be important to maintain a consistent record to understand if you are seeing any positive results through the use of the diet.

Outcomes

One important thing to note here is that, the results of the diet will vary from person to person. It will not be the same for all people and so it is important to understand that the results will come through depending on your body type and the amount of fat that is present in your body and particularly, your belly. So do not compare yourself with others and do not give up on the diet. Your progress might be slow but once you start to see the results, you will be able to accelerate your weight loss and attain a healthy and slim body.

Children

Although the diet is meant for obese children as well, it is best that a physician be consulted. Many children will need to be on a normal diet despite being fat, as their bodies will need extra nutrition to grow. If your child is morbidly obese, then you can take up the diet but if he/ she can reduce the weight through exercise, then it is best they take up activities such as swimming, cycling etc.

Pregnant women

Pregnant women, like children, might need some extra nutrition and most are not allowed to go on a fatty diet. So it is best that these consult a physician first, as the diet might have a bearing on the unborn child. The diet might also cause a new mother to not produce enough milk and so, it is best that she consult a physician first.

Side effects

If the ketogenic diet is not followed properly then conditions such as liver and kidney damage can occur. They might occur owing to excess secretion of ketones, which contain chemicals such as acetone and benzophenone, which might cause damage to these organs if not transported to the brain.

Apart from these, temporary side effects such as nausea, dizziness and sugar cravings may occur, but these do not last long and as soon as the body gets adjusted to the diet, they will disappear.

These form the warnings and precautions of the ketogenic diet and it is important for you to know that these are just statutory warnings and must not deter you from taking up the diet.

Low Carb

Chapter 4: Understanding the Benefits of Ketogenic Diets

Part one of this book, has given you a basic outline of the principles of the Ketogenic Diet, as well as all the information you need to get you started – the good stuff, the things to watch out for, and some recipes to get you started. By now, you should be getting into the swing of low carb dieting, and losing some of that excess weight. You should also be feeling better about your body.

Knowledge is power, as the saying goes, so now it's time to look deeper into low carb diets, because it's easy to get complacent, especially when you're seeing speedy results. However, if you have a lot of weight to lose, you're going to be looking at a long term plan, and the more you know about low carb dieting, the more you can adapt it to suit your lifestyle, so you never get bored or feel deprived. To motivate you even more, let's look at the benefits of low carb dieting.

Keeps you fuller for longer

Low carb diets are also high protein diets, and protein is Nature's filler. Protein foods can be very satisfying, and they also take longer to digest, which means the metabolism works harder, using up more calories in the process. These are calories that could end up stored as fat, so your body benefits in two ways from a low carb diet.

Lean proteins such as eggs, poultry and fish are also lower in calories than carbohydrates, so you don't need so many calories to keep hunger pains at bay. And remember that beans and other legumes are high in protein too, so it doesn't always have to be meat for your main protein choices. Remember to trim excess fat off meat, and cook your proteins with little or no added fat, because calories still count, and fat is very high in calories.

More filling power means you're more likely to stick with the diet, and your calorie deficit will be greater, so that means there's also more potential for weight loss.

Fast weight loss

Because low carb diets are also filling, they are also easier to stick to, which means that people who have failed in previous attempts to lose weight may be able to succeed with a low carb diet. Low carb is particularly helpful for people with big appetites, those with a lot of weight to lose, or people who don't feel they've had a meal unless there's a good helping of protein on the plate.

Various studies have shown that it's possible to lose two or three times as much weight on a low carb diet compared with more traditional low fat diets. These benefits are particularly evident during the first six months of dieting, and this is the crucial time.

In the early stages of weight loss, it's possible to get de-motivated and even give up if, after a week of sticking religiously to the eating plan and feeling hungry for most of that week, you haven't lost any weight at all.

Low carb diets also rid the body of excess sodium, which tends to retain water and make for an uncomfortable, bloated feeling. This helps to achieve spectacular weight loss in those crucial, make-or-break early weeks.

Effective for losing visceral fat

When people say they want to lose weight, what they really mean is that they want to lose fat. And when they want to lose fat what they really mean is that they want to lose belly fat. And this is where low carb and ketogenic diets come into their own, because you're likely to lose more belly fat on low carb and ketogenic diets than any other.

As well as looking unsightly, those rolls of fat around your middle are also dangerous to your health, and here's why. There are two types of body fat – subcutaneous fat, which lie beneath the skin, and visceral fat, which is deeper seated and tends to gather around the organs. Most of the body's organs are situated in the abdomen, so it follows that most of the fat in that area is visceral fat.

The problem with visceral fat is that you can't see it, so you don't realize how big the problem is, until you are hit by something like diabetes, cardiovascular disease or even some forms of cancer. Visceral fat contributes to internal inflammation, and that is at the root of many chronic health conditions.

Low carb diets are great for losing fat, and most of it is visceral fat, so it's the most dangerous type of fat health wise. Visceral fat also causes metabolic problems, and that interferes with weight loss and the body's natural hormonal balance.

Lowers triglycerides and raises HDL cholesterol levels

Most people know that high levels of 'good' high-density lipoprotein (HDL) cholesterol are good for cardiovascular health, but that's just one side of the story. Triglycerides are also part of the picture. These are also blood fats, and if your triglyceride levels are high, your HDL cholesterol levels will be dropping to an unhealthy level.

In blood tests, the ratio of triglycerides to HDL cholesterol is a good risk indicator for cardiovascular problems and diabetes, and some experts believe that high triglyceride levels can be more problematic than high 'bad' LDL cholesterol. High triglyceride levels are usually due to an unhealthy lifestyle – being overweight, smoking, not getting enough exercise and eating a lot of processed foods and foods high in sugar all contribute to the problem.

Why do they call HDL 'good' cholesterol while LDL is the bad guy? Basically, it's down to the way they work in the body. LDL transports cholesterol out of the liver and around the body, and therein lies the problem. Too much LDL clogs the arteries, leaving you vulnerable to heart disease. HDL carries cholesterol from the body to the liver, therefore removing the risk. Once safely lodged in the liver, the cholesterol can be excreted or repurposed.

So, if low carb diets raise HDL and lower triglycerides, it's a win-win situation. It's the higher proportion of healthy dietary fats that achieves this happy state of affairs. Low fat diets tend to raise triglyceride and HDL cholesterol levels.

Lowers blood sugar levels

Of the three macronutrients – proteins, carbohydrates and fats – only carbohydrates actually increase blood sugar levels. Protein raises levels slightly; fat has no impact. This means that proteins and fats do not encourage insulin production. And that means a low carb diet leaves you at less risk of developing diabetes.

When the body produces too much insulin, it doesn't burn fat effectively, so that stops you losing weight. With low fat diets, there's the risk that the body will burn muscle tissue rather than fat to provide the energy your body needs to function properly. By reducing your carbohydrate intake, you restore the insulin balance in your body and regularize blood sugar levels, and it all happens fairly quickly too.

Okay, it's possible to control blood sugar levels with medication, but all medications have some side effects, so if you can do this naturally it's so much better. One of the side effects with such medication is weight gain, and that's likely to add to your problems, rather than solving them.

Lowering your carbohydrate intake works better than medication, because it's a more natural and efficient process. In fact it's so efficient that if you are already on medication to lower your blood sugar levels, you need to keep an eye on things, or you could end up hypoglycemic. However, many physicians and nutritionists agree that the majority of people can benefit from reducing the amount of insulin in their bodies. And the best way to do this is to reduce your carbohydrate intake with a low carb diet.

With so many health advantages to low carbohydrate diets, one has to wonder why some people are so set against them. It has to be said that this way of eating may not suit everyone, and it's not thought to be so effective in the long term. However, if you raise your carb intake gradually once you reach target weight, you can monitor any increases and deal with it before it gets out of hand. Learn as much as you can about the system, because after all, knowledge is power!

Chapter 5: Exercising on a Low Carbohydrate Diet

While it's difficult to get a consensus from nutrition and fitness experts on the effectiveness and safety of low carb and ketogenic diets, one thing everyone seems to agree on is that diet alone – whatever program you follow – is not enough to help you to lose weight and keep it off. You need some exercise in your life to tone and firm your body, build muscle mass and keep you lean.

Exercise boosts the metabolism, so it will also help you to lose excess weight more quickly. How does that work? Well, exercise builds muscle, and muscle mass burns calories at around 3 times the rate of fat cells. Each pound of muscle burns around 6 calories per day, while a pound of fat burns 2 calories in the same time frame. If that doesn't seem a lot, multiply it out over the days in the year, and that equates to quite a lot of fat burning power over the year.

A word of caution though. Because carbohydrates provide energy, you need to rethink your workout routine, as clearly on a low carb diet your energy levels are going to be depleted. Also, you are taking in fewer calories, and the body is programmed to find the missing energy from somewhere, in order to keep you going. So, you have to structure your workout so you get maximum benefit without depleting your energy stores so that you feel really tired and your muscles are sore.

It's worth it, though, because exercise raises your core body temperature, and depresses your appetite. You know how on a hot summer day you don't feel like eating much? Well, it's the same after a good exercise session, so it's a double benefit. Not only are you using calories by exercising, you're saving calories at mealtimes too. It's a win-win situation.

Short intense workouts are best on a low carb diet, so if you have a heavy afternoon booked at the gym, cancel it right now. In fact you don't really need to do the gym at all – you can get all the exercise you need without even going through the doors of a gym. An hour's session in the gym uses about 400- 500 calories an hour and you can easily work of those calories with brisk exercise.

Building up to walking

Briskly walking a mile burns 100 calories, and you should be able to walk 4 miles in an hour, so there are your 400 gym calories. If you find yourself tiring easily, start off with short burst of walking, to give your body chance to adapt to your low-carb eating plan.

Research has shown that it doesn't matter how short your walks are, if you put the effort in, the results are the same. So, if you don't have the time for a 30-minute walk, fit in six five-minute walks, or even 10 three-minute walks. The end benefit will be exactly the same. However, if you're going down the 'bite-sized walk' route, you need to be meticulous about the timing, to ensure that you're doing enough brisk walking to get the full benefits.

Swimming

Swimming is great exercise – its high intensity aerobic exercise, and it uses just about every major muscle group in the body. It can also burn up the calories, and combined with a low carb diet, it will soon get rid of your excess body fat. Half an hour of vigorous swimming burns between at least 350 calories, depending on the strokes you use.

However, you need to adjust your eating patterns to ensure you have enough energy to swim for long enough to make a difference. The best way to do this is to schedule one third of your carb allowance around an hour before your swim to give you an energy boost. Eat another third right afterwards to help with recovery, and spread the rest of your carbs through the day.

This is a good strategy to apply on any day where you're likely to be doing any kind of high intensity aerobic exercise. Your muscles need a glycogen boost to help them work through your training session, and dividing up your carbs in this way will give them that boost.

However, if you'd rather not take that approach, why not fit in your exercise session immediately after waking? The body's natural insulin levels are low at this time, and some experts are of the opinion that this accelerates fat burning. The thing is, everyone is different, and so you may need to experiment to find the exercise routine that works best for you in conjunction with your low carb diet.

Above all, your exercise should be something you enjoy. If you enjoy the gym, that's fine – exercise at the gym. It doesn't need to be all machine exercise – you can perform squats, lunges and jump squats in between sessions on the apparatus to change up the activity and make it a little easier on your muscles. Whether it's swimming, walking, cycling, dancing or any other form of exercise, if you enjoy doing it, you're more likely to stick with it, so settle on something you enjoy.

Forget anything you may have heard about low carb diets only being good for people who lead sedentary lives. The human body was never designed to be sedentary – it was designed to move, but as a species we've become sedentary, and that needs to change if you're serious about losing weight and getting fit.

Chapter 6: Exploding the Myths about Low Carbohydrate and Ketogenic Diets

There's so much written about low carb and ketogenic diets, it can all get confusing. The problem is, low carb polarizes opinion. People are either very much for it, or very much against it, and there's nothing in between. For the person new to this type of dieting, it's helpful to explode some of the myths, and set the record straight.

One thing to remember is that everybody is an individual, and everybody is different in its composition and tolerance for various foods and exercise routines. All sorts of things play a part in this – heredity, general health, build, and personal preference. No diet can ever be 'one size fits all' simply because no two people are alike, and while low carb dieting is very effective for some people, others may not be able to get the results they want and may even become ill on it.

That doesn't mean there's anything wrong with the diet or the person – it's just the way it is. Here are some of the more persistent and pernicious myths about low carbohydrate and ketogenic diets.

Low carb diets are the best

As mentioned in the introduction, low carb diets are not a good fit for everyone, even though it is one of the most effective ways to lose surplus weight quickly without feeling hungry or deprived.

However, due to the many differences between individuals, low carb eating is not a universal plan. People with insulin resistance can certainly benefit from low carb eating, because it damps down insulin production and boosts insulin sensitivity. This means the body is able to maintain healthy levels of insulin and regulate blood sugar levels without the need for medication. This makes low carb eating a suitable way to lose weight for people with type-2 diabetes, as long as they work under medical supervision. Indeed, anyone with a chronic health condition should not embark on any new eating plan without the consent and supervision of their medical advisors.

People with gluten intolerance or celiac disease may also benefit from a low carb diet, which is naturally low in gluten, but again medical advice is important. Also, people with fatty livers can benefit from low carb eating, since when carbs are restricted, the liver produces less LDL cholesterol. This allows the body to burn more of the stored fat, since production is damped down.

If you have a tendency towards constipation and some digestive orders, low carb dieting could exacerbate these problems, as low carb diets tend to be lower in fiber than more vegetable-based diets such as the Mediterranean Diet. People with hypothyroidism (underactive thyroid) may also find that low carb eating is unsuitable for them, since carbohydrates encourage thyroid stimulating hormone production to balance activity. Low carb eating could in this instance cause further metabolic problems.

Professional athletes, or just those who exercise for several hours a day on a regular basis, may also find that low carb eating affects their performance and increases recovery time. It may still be possible to work on a restricted carb plan, without going too low, but talk it over with your trainer and nutritionist.

We really can't emphasize this enough – check with your physician before embarking on a low carb diet. Although it's generally a healthy way to eat, there may be contraindications for some people, and your health professional is the best person to advice on this.

All carbs are fattening

Let's get this straight – any foods are fattening if you eat more than your body requires, because the excess is stored as fat. Don't think in terms of calories here – think of sugar content when you're sorting the good carbs from the bad. Refined carbohydrates are always going to be high in sugar and fat – white bread, rice and pasta, cakes and cookies – so these are the carbs to eliminate from your diet.

Asian diets are very high carbohydrate, as they are based around rice – even at breakfast time. However, you don't see many Asians who need to lose weight, so that should prove that carbs are not necessarily fattening if you make the right choices and avoid frying your carbs.

Make your carb choices from the complex carbohydrates that have been through little or no processing. Go for whole meal bread, brown rice, and whole-wheat pasta. And monitor the quantities carefully. All diets work because you consume fewer calories than your body needs, forcing it to burn fat stores in order to function normally, so portion control is important, whatever diet you're following.

Instead of thinking of specific foods and food groups as fattening, train yourself to think of foods as healthy or unhealthy, natural or processed. Opt for natural foods, and cook from scratch, so you avoid hidden fats and sugars. It may surprise you to know that even low calorie, tomato-based pasta sauces contain significant amounts of sugar, to preserve the sauce and improve flavor and color.

Check out the nutrition labels, but better yet, batch cook your own healthy foods and freeze them for future use. Ultimately, it's cheaper and healthier, and you are in full control of what goes into your body.

Avoid fruits, carrots and potatoes

This is probably the most dangerous of all the low carb myths out there. The reason it gains traction is because these foods contain carbohydrates, but the thing to remember is the diet is LOW carb not NO carb. If you eliminate a complete food group from your diet, you are asking for major health problems, and sooner rather than later. Carbohydrates are one of the three macronutrients, along with proteins and fats, and while a low carb diet restricts your intake of these foods, it's really about eliminating unhealthy carbs and making choices from the many healthy carbs available.

Fruits, potatoes and carrots may contain carbohydrates, but they have other health benefits too, and a sensible low carb diet is all about weighing the carb content against the other nutritional advantages and disadvantages.

Fruit is a good example here. Yes, there is carbohydrate in there, but fruits are a great source of antioxidants and vitamins – especially the brightly colored varieties. Antioxidants are vital for boosting the immune system and fighting the free radicals that encourage premature aging and are thought to cause a number of cancers. The carb content comes from fructose, which of course is sugar, but it's a natural sugar, unlike the refined sugars that go into the production of that pasta sauce we were talking about earlier. It's the same with carrots and potatoes.

One vital thing that these carb-containing foods provide is fiber. Low carb diets do tend to be a little low on fiber, which can cause constipation and digestive problems for some people, but if you include these foods in your diet, you'll be getting a good dose of fiber. And as long as you cook them without fat, they're pretty low in calories too. Remember – it's not just about the carb count – calories and portion control is important if you're going to lose weight on a low carb diet.

Low carb and ketogenic diets are the same animal

A lot if the 'anti' feeling surrounding low carb diets arises because people wrongly assume that low carb and ketogenic are interchangeable terms – even synonyms. This is just not true.

A low carb diet is exactly that – low in carbohydrates. 'Low' varies, depending on the individual concerned. It can mean anything from 50 to 150 grams of carbohydrate per day, or even more in some cases. Normal nutritional recommendations suggest that 45 – 65% of your daily calories should come from carbohydrate sources. That's somewhere between 900 and 1300 for most people, or around 225 – 325 daily carb grams for someone eating 2000 calories a day.

A ketogenic diet is very low in carbohydrates – the aim is for less than 50 grams per day, to induce a state of ketosis. That's a process whereby lowering the intake of carbohydrates deprives the body of glucose needed for energy, forcing it to burn fat stores instead. It can be beneficial for people with metabolic syndrome, and kick start weight loss in severely obese people without causing feelings of hunger. However, while low carb diets are not necessarily high in fat, the ketogenic diet derives around 75% of its calories from fat, with just 20% coming from proteins, and the remaining 5% from carbohydrates.

Some medical professionals see this as a dangerous way to diet, because it severely restricts one of the macronutrients, while encouraging people to consume more than twice the recommended daily allowance of fats.

Carbs and sugars are not always the same

It gets a bit confusing when people generalize by saying that all carbs are broken down into sugar in the body, and that all carbs contain sugar. Mention sugars to most people, and they think of the white granulated stuff that goes in coffee and on cornflakes. However, it's not that simple, and neither is the way the body processes carbohydrates to extract substances it can use to fuel the body's essential functions.

There are numerous forms of sugar – sucrose, fructose, lactose, and dextrose – to name but a few, and you probably need a degree in chemistry to understand exactly how each sugar works in the body. Simply put, the body uses glucose, which is a starch extracted from sugar, to provide energy and keep the muscles healthy. Talking of glucose as a sugar is confusing the issue, and basically saying that a potato – which is a healthy and filling form of carbohydrate – is in the same camp as an unhealthy, blood sugar elevating candy bar. That's probably all you need to know to get the most benefit from your low carb diet, so don't sweat the rest of it.

You won't gain weight by eating low carb

This myth is probably responsible for most of the bad press low carb diets get. A lot of this arises from the simple fact that people tend to overlook – any diet, whether it says so in the rules or not, will only help you to lose weight if you are eating fewer calories than your body is using to function. In order to lose one pound in weight, you need to consume 3,500 less calories than your body needs. This is undisputable science, and you can't walk away from it.

If your normal daily calorie intake is 2,000, and you want to lose 1lb per week from January 1 until your vacation in April so you can fit into a tiny bikini on the beach, you are going to have to reduce your calorie intake to 1,500 a day – every day. If you take all those calories as chocolate, or all of them as lettuce, you will lose that prized pound every week, although nobody rather than a lunatic would recommend that you did such a thing. We're just using this example to show that calorie restriction is the only way to lose weight, whatever fancy name a particular diet may go by.

Some of the foods that are unrestricted on low carb diets are also very high in fat and calories – cheese, butter, cream, peanut butter, oils, nuts – all need to be portion controlled and calorie counted if you're going to keep your daily totals low enough to lose weight. The sensible thing to do is maximize your calorie benefit so that you get the most filling power from the fewest calories. That means going for lean fish, poultry, and eggs and lean meats, and keeping the really high calorie stuff for treats and snacks, rather than eating them as main meals.

Because low carb eating naturally dumbs down your appetite due to the protein and complex carbohydrates, you're automatically going to be restricting your calorie intake anyway, and you may get away without counting calories, if your judgment of portion size is pretty good. However, if you're not losing weight on a low carb diet, it's most likely because you're serving up too much high calorie stuff, or being over generous on portion size for the healthier food items. Be honest about this, and try weighing portions for a few days to see if that makes a difference.

Just because a food item is unrestricted on a particular diet plan, it doesn't mean you can indulge to your heart's content. That's what made you overweight in the first place, and it's not going to help you to lose weight. You need to educate yourself regarding calories and nutrition. It's easier to count calories on a low carb diet, but you still need to put in the effort to get the results. There is no 'quick fix' for weight loss. You didn't get fat overnight, and you won't get your figure back without working on it either.

Fiber doesn't matter

Because low carb dieting also means low fiber eating, some people assume that fiber is not important. However, nothing could be further from the truth. Fiber in the diet is essential – without it, you'll suffer constipation, digestive problems and elevated cholesterol levels.

The mistake people make is thinking that there is only one kind of fiber, like they think there's only one kind of sugar. Soluble fiber helps with weight loss, because it helps you to feel fuller for longer for a modest calorie count. Also, fiber helps to lower cholesterol levels in the blood and protect against heart disease. Your body needs fiber to stay healthy, so don't assume that it's not important, just because it's not such a major player in low carb diets.

Carbs cause health problems

Low carb diets have been very successful in treating some disorders, particularly those associated with the metabolism, such as diabetes and metabolic syndrome. That leads some people to conclude that if low carb eating makes you better, then eating a high carb diet must have made you ill, so carbs are the enemy of good health and long life.

Nothing could be further from the truth, actually. Carbs didn't make you ill – genetic factors and lifestyle choices did that for you. Restricting carbs can have dramatic effects on health, mainly because it regulates the body's production of insulin, and stabilizes blood sugar levels.

However, if you've been paying attention so far, you've realized that not all carbohydrates are created equal. Refined carbohydrates are high in fats and sugars, and can create the blood sugar spikes that make you crave even more of those unhealthy foods. They're also highly processed, with hidden ingredients like fats, sugars and salt that are the enemies of healthy eating. So, it's not the carbohydrates that are the problem, it's the carbohydrates you choose to include in your diet. There's a big difference.

The thing with low carb diets, as we've said before, is that they polarize opinion, and people make too many wrong assumptions, based on what they think they know about low carb eating. It's healthy, and it works – but not for everyone. And you need to understand how basic nutrition works in order to fully understand why low carb diets work, and why they might not work if you don't take on board all the principles of low carb dieting.

When people see a diet that seems to allow them to eat lots of food and still lose weight, they tend to fix on the headline points and ignore the nitty gritty, and that's when it can all go spectacularly wrong. Then people blame the diet, when they should be looking in the mirror for reasons for failure. The first requirement of any weight loss diet is honesty, and that can only come from you.

Chapter 7: Advantages and disadvantages of Going Ketogenic

As explained previously, ketogenic and low carb diets are two different things, although they share some similarities. Low carb means taking in 50 – 150 grams of carbohydrate a day, rather than the recommended 225 – 325 grams for a normal healthy diet. Ketogenic involves very low levels of carbohydrates – less than 50 grams per day – and is also high fat, since around 75% of each day's calories are derived from fats, with 20% coming from proteins and just 5% from carbohydrates. Low carb diets are not necessarily high in either protein or fat.

The purpose of ketogenic dieting is to induce a state of ketosis in the body. This occurs when the body does not have enough glucose to convert to energy to fuel normal bodily functions. The body is then forced burn stored fat to make up the energy requirements, since the very low level of carbohydrate intake means glucose is in short supply.

As with any eating plan, ketogenic dieting has its aficionados and detractors. It is certainly a more extreme form of dieting – one which all except the most motivated people may find difficult to stay with. Here's a summary of the advantages and disadvantages of ketogenic diets, to help you decide if you want to take that extra step in order to lose those excess pounds.

Advantages

More dramatic fat loss: When ketosis occurs as a result of extremely low carbohydrate intake, the body is forced to burn its fat stores for energy, in addition to metabolizing that fat you take in every day. Because the body is programmed to store fat in case of famine, it can be very difficult to persuade it to part with those precious fat stores, but ketogenic dieting can achieve the almost impossible, and coerce the body into using its fat stores, particularly when the diet is paired with an effective exercise program.

Management of epilepsy and improved brain health: Originally, ketogenic diets were developed back in the 1920s to help manage epilepsy, particularly in children. During ketosis, molecules called ketones are produced, and these are believed to alter the brain chemistry, so that seizures are controlled and may even cease altogether. Recent research suggests that the ketogenic diet may even be helpful in preventing the onset of Alzheimer's disease in adults, or at least managing the disease.

Reduced risk of cancer: It's well known that everybody has cancer cells within them – they just need the perfect storm of physical conditions to develop into the full works. Cancer cells need sugar to live to fight another day; therefore, severely restricting carbs deprives them of what they need most. While most of the body's cells can adapt to use whatever is available for them at the time, cancer cells haven't worked out how to make Ketones work to their advantage, so the cells will die off. If you are eating a super healthy diet, it is another kick in the teeth for those pesky cancer cells.

So, effectively, there are three powerful advantages to following a ketogenic diet. However, that is a pretty small list, so maybe it's time to check out the disadvantages before committing to a very low carb diet.

Disadvantages

May compromise a very active lifestyle: One criticism of regular low carb dieting is that it may leave active people such as those with physically demanding jobs and athletes with depleted energy levels which may compromise performance and recovery. When it comes to ketogenic dieting, the problem is magnified considerably.

Difficult to stick to: While there is a certain level of flexibility in low carb eating plans, ketogenic diets are much more restrictive, and this can prove a problem when socializing or eating in college or work place restaurants. If you're inducing ketosis for weight loss, you may be more tempted to cheat, simply because so many foods are forbidden on this diet plan, and the ratio of fat to carbohydrate is high.

May be harmful to health: A ketogenic diet is good for fat loss, but the high fat content means you're at increased risk of heart disease. This creates a nutritional paradox, because losing weight is supposed to lower the risk of heart disease, while eating high levels of fat increases it. It's difficult to pinpoint the exact point at which the disadvantages of ketosis outweigh the benefits.

Can cause permanent damage to the metabolism: In the short term, a ketogenic diet shifts body fat by forcing the body to burn its jealously guarded fat stores in order to provide the energy needed for normal bodily function. However, in the long run, very low carbohydrate consumption can irrevocably damage the metabolism. The ironic thing is that a certain amount of carbohydrate is necessary to keep the muscles hydrated. When muscles are adequately hydrated, the metabolism stays raised, because it thinks the body is well fed, and there is no need to slow down to conserve energy. This needs to be understood if you are aiming to lose fat without destroying muscle tone. Remember that muscles burn 6 calories per pound per day, while fat burns just two calories per pound per day, so it's worth getting that balance right.

On the face of it, there are more disadvantages than advantages in following a ketogenic diet. However, as we have said before, everyone is different, both in mental make up and physiology, so whatever diet you are following, you need to adapt it to suit your personal circumstances and lifestyle. Enlist the help of a nutritionist and a personal trainer to get the balance right for weight loss and improved muscle tone, without compromising the metabolism in increasing the risk of heart disease.

Ketosis works, but it needs to be closely managed by people who fully understand the principles and the pitfalls. It's not something you go into unprepared, so take the time to read up about it and get expert help. And it goes without saying; if you have any chronic health conditions, check with your physician before embarking on the ketogenic diet so that he can advise you, based on your current health situation.

Low Carb

Chapter 8: The Mistakes that May Prevent You Losing Weight on a Low Carb Diet

If you've read everything so far, you've probably come to the conclusion that low carb dieting is a great way to lose weight and burn off fat, and you'd be right. However, although it's a fairly straightforward way to weight loss, you need to know what you're doing and why, because if you get it wrong, you may not lose weight, and could even end up gaining pounds.

That's soul destroying, so here's a roundup of the common mistakes people make when following a low carb diet. Forewarned is forearmed, so make sure you don't fall victim to any of these diet destroyers. And remember, it's not all about the numbers on the scales, as the first point proves. Some of the things you see, as failures in the diet may just be misconceptions on your part so don't lose faith. You can do it – and you will!

Weighing in too often

This is a big mistake in any diet, because weight fluctuates by the hour, and it can be very demoralizing when you know you've had a good dieting day, but the scales disagree with you. However, because of the unique physical changes that occur on low carb diets, it's particularly important not to place too much reliance on the numbers.

If you need a measure of success, try measuring for inch loss, or trying on clothes that were previously too tight. If you're sticking to the low carb regime, controlling portion size and keeping an eye on calories, as well as including some exercise each day, you are definitely losing fat – which is what we really mean when we say we want to lose weight.

Use the way you look and the way you feel as your success indicators, rather than what the scales say. Because your fat store is going down, your ratio of muscle mass will be increasing, especially if you are exercising, and while increased muscle mass may initially show as a slight weight gain, in the long run, the more muscle you have, the better you look and the faster your metabolism, so you will reap the rewards – just be a little patient.

Still eating processed food

We've already mentioned that processed food often contains hidden sugars that may be messing around with your carefully calculated carb count. The way out of this problem is to cook from scratch, and buy natural foods. If you don't recognize it, don't buy it, and don't eat it.

Even those so-called healthy low carb snacks can mess around with your body if you're particularly sensitive to carbohydrates.

It's not that there's anything wrong with them or with you – just that they don't suit you. If you can honestly say that you're following the low carb diet, but still not losing weight or inches, maybe you need to completely exorcise processed foods from your meal plans.

Think you don't have time to cook from scratch? Bulk cook simple stuff like pasta sauces, soups and low carb meals and freeze them for later use. In the long run, it's healthier and cheaper. Treat yourself to some hot new clothes with the money you save.

Eating too much high calorie food

When you're eating a low carb diet, it's easy to eat too much high protein and high calorie food without even realizing it. Foods such as nuts and full fat dairy products are high in protein, but also high in calories and fats, and unless you're checking out those portions, you could be in for a nasty shock when you step on the scales. You need to get the balance right between calories, proteins, carbs and fats if you're going to lose weight on a low carb diet plan.

Too much dairy can also cause insulin spikes, which messes about with your metabolism, and can stop you from reaping the full benefits of a low carb diet, and there's more sugar than you might think in some yogurts. You really do need to take a long hard look at everything you eat, not just the carbs – seriously!

Thinking it's all about the carbs

The big mistake people make on low carb diets is thinking all they need to do is adjust their carb intake and the weight will just fall off. It's just not as simple as that – the science behind low carb dieting is straightforward enough, but you need to be up to speed with it if you're going to lose weight the low carb way.

The way you're eating – if you're doing it right - forces your metabolism to change, so that you burn off excess fat. However, if you're taking in too many calories, or eating too much protein, or not enough fat, you'll upset the balance.

Too much animal protein can cause the amino acids to turn into glucose, and that can mess up your diet. Aim to eat no more than 1.5 – 2 grams of protein per kilo of body weight per day. So, if you weigh 70 kilos, you're looking at 105 – 140 grams of protein on a very low carb diet aimed at achieving ketosis.

Another mistake people make is thinking that pairing low fat dieting with low carb dieting will bring even better results. That really isn't so – if you're not eating carbs, you need to give your body something to take fuel from and give you energy. And the best way to do this is to eat more fats. If you're following a ketogenic diet, around 70 – 75% of your daily calorie intake should come from fat. You need something to replace the carbs you ditched, otherwise it is not going to be pretty – and neither are you.

The thing about low carb and ketogenic dieting is that it's flexible, so you can plan your diet around your lifestyle. However, you do need to understand how the diet works, and why it is important to do the things you do. If you don't know how your metabolism works, you won't know how to kick start it to give yourself a big weight loss boost at the start of the diet, so this isn't a diet for wimps. However, you can achieve spectacular results if you can get the balance between proteins, carbs, fats and calories just right.

It's not easy, but then nothing worth having ever is, is it? And this is worth having, because done right, this diet can deplete your fat stores quicker than just about any other. In addition, it can reduce your chances of developing heart disease, diabetes, and even some cancers in later life. What's not to love? Get into the groove of low carb dieting, and award yourself the body you deserve. You know it makes sense!

Chapter 9: The Importance of Exercise

Benefits of regular physical activity

Regular exercise and physical activity are essential for proper maintenance of health. However, exercise is more than just about health as it has several benefits apart from health maintenance. Regular exercise has the potential to improve your mood as well as enhance your sex life. This chapter will revolve around the various ways that exercise can improve your life

No matter how hard you try to stay away from exercise, the advantages that regular physical activities possess are hard to ignore. One of the major benefits of exercise is that it is non-discriminating, as it does not discriminate on the basis of age, physical ability or gender.

Weight control

Exercise has the unique ability to maintain your weight or assist in your weight loss. This is because you burn calories when you exercise. If you go for higher-intensity exercises, the calories you burn will be far greater. Moreover, for effective weight loss you will not have to allocate time separately for exercise as they can be done in a short span of time or in your daily chores (in climbing stairs etc.)

Fighting Diseases

If you're majorly bothered by health conditions like heart disease or high blood pressure, exercising will help you prevent their development. Physical activities increase the concentration of high-density lipoprotein (HDL), which is commonly known as 'good cholesterol' and decreases the concentration of unhealthy triglycerides. They also promote efficient blood flow from the body to the heart and vice-versa, reducing the chances of development of cardiovascular diseases. Exercise helps your body fight against stroke, depression, cancer, arthritis; metabolic syndrome, type II diabetes.

Better mood

Exercise is ideal if you need to blow off some steam or find a way to release accumulated stress from work. A 30-minute walk can give you a much-needed emotional lift. This is because exercise and physical activity stimulate the secretion of various proteins, which eliminate toxins from your brain, thereby leaving you with a much happier and more relaxed feel.

Better sleep

If you experience irregular sleep patterns, physical activity is the right way to spend your time. As you progress into your exercise, your body will feel exhausted which will help you fall asleep faster. However, if your exercises just before you go to bed, your body will be in an energized state, which will delay your sleep.

An enhanced sex life

If you feel you lack physical intimacy, it is because of your lack of physical activity. If you exercise regularly your body feels energized and also looks better and not clumsy, which has a positive influence on your sex life? It has been found that regular exercise counteracts the development of various sexual problems seen in men like erectile dysfunction or premature ejaculation.

Fun

Exercise is an ideal way to kill time while having fun. It offers you the chance to relax and enjoy the surroundings around you by engaging you in activities, which make you, feel comfortable and happy. A physical activity like a dance class or a sport will help you connect with people and improve your interpersonal skills.

Exercising and physical activity is a great way to not only enjoy the health benefits but also to have fun. It is always recommended you start slow and focus only on 30 minutes of physical activity every day. If you have particular fitness goals, you will have to alter the intensity of your workout. Consult your physician or doctor before you start exercising, especially if you aren't experienced to it or have certain health issues, which can serve as a barrier to your physical development.

Brian Adams

Chapter 10: Exercises to Overcome Belly Fat

In the previous chapter, we explored the potential and importance of physical activity for maintenance of health. Having established that, it's important to know about the different exercises you could practice for reducing your belly fat.

Most people relate reducing belly fat to the development of an 'ab'. 'Ab/Abs' are more than just a muffin top and are formally known as abdominals, collectively forming a core network of several interconnected muscles that span the entire course of your back and then stretch around your butt and the front and inner thighs.

For developing your abdominal region, your exercises should focus mainly on getting more from your core. Be it through Pilates, Yoga, or through core-focused exercises. Before you begin the exercises, you must follow certain tips for a better outcome thereby enhancing your activity.

- Move your waist. As you twist your body, ensure that the movement is consistent from your bottom rib. It is also recommended you keep your hips still.

- Be firm. It is mandatory that during each exercise, your body is tight and erect forming a sharp angle. You should get a similar feeling as you do when wearing tight jeans, precisely at the point of one hipbone to the other.

- Take deep breaths. This is a quite popular tip while doing any form of physical activity as it calms the senses. However, while exercising it strengthens the bed for development of your 'ab/abs' and aids your lower back. With every deep breath, remember to exhale just as thoroughly

Here are some of the best exercises that you may want to try.

A new kind of crunch

This exercise is popularly referred to as the two-in-one abs-and-obliques move. It's a simple exercise; firstly you'll have to sit in a manner so that your thighs and upper torso are together forming a V while lifting your lower legs and crossing them slightly.

Hold a 5-pound dumbbell (or a ball of equal proportion) between both hands. Turn gently from left to right and vice versa, and move the ball with you while retaining the V shape.

3 sets of 15 reps with a frequency of 3–4 times a week are recommended.

Bridge and opposite arm to leg reach

This exercise was made popular by countless fitness experts and is extremely useful for taking the inches from your waistline. It is also a move which can be practiced anywhere anytime.

Firstly, lie down with your face facing the roof and bend your left knee. In this position, maintain your left foot towards the floor. Extend your right leg as far as possible in the direction of the ceiling. Similarly, extend your left arm towards the ceiling and keep your right arm on the floor.

After holding this position, move the raised leg to the right and the raised arm to the left, while keeping your hips or shoulders still. Shifting your focus to the abs, return your raised leg and arm to the original position.

One round each of 10–12 reps for each side every day is recommended.

Low-belly leg reach

This exercise has the ability to develop your corset and six-pack. It will have you lie down facing the ceiling while bending your knees to a complete 90 degrees, hands behind your head, with your abs contracted. Stack your knees over your hips while lifting your shoulders to crunch them up. Hold this position for 3-5 seconds and inhale a deep breath.

Exhale and stretch your legs to form a 45-degree angle. Hold this position for another 3-5 seconds and put pressure on your lower belly.

Two sets of this exercise each day for around 10-15 reps is ideal.

Teaser

Consider this exercise as an advanced Pilates-inspired move. You'll have to lie with your face towards the ceiling and bend your knees to form a 90-degree angle with your body and feet. Inhale deeply and tighten your abdominal region. As you inhale, lift your arms and put them back over your head.

As you exhale, swing your arms forward and stretch your legs so as to form a V. As this exercise is comparatively harder, you can take the aid of your hands by placing them for additional support.

After you exhale, roll down slowly and retain your original position.

15 reps of this exercise daily are recommended.

Donkey kickbacks

This exercise is popular among most physical trainers as it has the ability to burn a lot of calories if done regularly and in the right way. You'll have to kneel on the floor with your toes tucked under your feet and your spine erect. Take your belly in toward your back and tighten your abdominal region. While doing so, lift your knees to an elevation of about 2 inches from the ground.

Keeping your abdominal region tight, extend your right knee to your nasal region. After this is done, kick your right leg behind you in a manner that your butt is pressured. To avoid pressurizing your back, ensure that your abdominal region is tight and the hips are facing the floor.

Repeat this procedure for around 8 times on each leg.

Advanced leg crunches

This exercise is prescribed for several celebrities who wish to make their body swimsuit ready in a shorter period of time.

Firstly, lie down facing the ceiling and bend your knees. Have someone place a 3-pound dumbbell between your feet and simultaneously rest your hands beneath your sitting bones with your palms facing the floor.

After this, focus on your lower abdominal region and utilize it to bring your knees towards your chest. While you're doing so, elevate your shoulders, hips, and head gradually. Immediately retain your original posture, completing 1 rep.

It is recommended you do a minimum of 15 or 30 reps with a frequency of 3–4 times every week. If done in the right way, the exercise is very effective and should produce positive results in less than 4 weeks.

The belly blaster

As indicated in the name, this exercise is very effective in busting your belly fat. This one is also known as Ana Caban's Belly blaster.

Firstly, you'll have to lie down with your face towards the ceiling while bending your knees and pushing them towards your chest. After attaining this posture, hold a 3-pound dumbbell in each hand. Stretch your left leg to form a 45-degree angle while bending your right knee. Lift your head and shoulders slightly, while you're doing this, move the dumbbells in your hands to the space above your right knee. Then press into a crunch. You can consider this as a second step.

Brian Adams

As a third step, try to get both your legs together so as to get your entire weight up towards the ceiling, while lifting your shoulders and head off the ground.

After this, repeat the second step, but this time around, switch to your left knee and so on, to complete one full rep.

Practice 8 such reps with a frequency of 4 times each week. If done effectively, you should see positive results within 3 weeks

Oblique driving-knee crunch

For this exercise, you'll have to lie down on a stability ball with your face towards the ceiling. When you're on the ball, ensure that the distance between your feet is approximately equal to the gap between your hips. While keeping your feet on the ground, bend your knees to form an angle of 90 degrees. After successfully bending your knees, place your right hand behind your head. For additional support, you can rest the palm of your left hand on the floor. Tighten your body's core region and lift your left foot off the floor up to a certain height, after this stretch the whole leg while keeping the foot flexed.

Consider this as a second step. While holding your previous posture, crunch your right shoulder and rib cage in towards your left knee, and stretch your right leg while keeping your foot on the ground. After this is done, retain your original posture with a stretched left leg and a bent right leg. This completes 1 rep.

Complete 15 reps on one side and then switch to the other side and repeat it for another 15.

Scale Pose

This exercise is a favorite among most people who hit the gym, as it is extremely efficient.

Firstly, you'll have to sit on a mat (or the floor) in a comfortable cross-legged posture with your hands adjacent to your hips. Pressurize your pelvic floor and tighten the entire area around it, and pump the energy you got to your hands and lift your entire lower body off the mat.

Hold this posture for 3 complete and deep breath cycles, and then gradually lower yourself. This exercise will challenge your strength, hence it is recommended for those who can't lift the lower half of their body completely to rest your feet on the ground and just elevate your butt.

3 reps of this exercise every day is recommended.

The Boat pose

For this exercise, you'll have to sit and bend your knees while your feet are resting on the ground and your hands are under your knees for balance. Lift your chest and shoulders back, while you're doing this tighten the region around your abs and lift your lower legs to a height where they are parallel to the ground. Ensure that your knees are entirely bent and your balance is intact.

If you are comfortable in this posture, you can proceed and straighten your legs and extend your arms forward. Once you've reached a position that is slightly out of your comfort zone, hold it for 5–15 deep breaths and then retain your original position.

Repeat this for approximately 5 times or so.

Cross-leg diagonal crunch
For this exercise, you'll have to lie down with your back on the ground while extending your legs and keeping your feet on the ground. Lift up your hips and shift them slightly towards the right while maintaining a still torso. Then slowly lower your hips and extend your legs in a similar manner as done earlier.

Next, you'll have to bend your left knee at an angle such that you can cross it over your right leg. While doing this, rest your left foot on the ground. After you have attained the posture, crunch upwards and gradually lower down.

50 reps of this exercise on either side are recommended.

Tone-it V Hold
This exercise mainly focuses on the delicate and flexible muscle fibers. These are responsible for contraction during exercises and help improve your muscular frame.

You'll have to sit on the floor and bend your knees while keeping your feet at ground level. Now, clasp the bottom side of your thighs with your hands, lean backward, and elevate your feet to a height where the lower part of your legs is parallel to ground level. In this position, release hands, extend your legs and touch the tip of your toes. If possible, hold the posture and take 8 deep breaths.

3 rounds of this exercise every day are recommended.

Plank
This exercise not only focuses on the entire core region but also has a significant influence in strengthening and tightening your arms, thighs, and butt.

For this exercise, you'll have to kneel down on a mat with your hands touching the surface of the mat forming a 90-degree angle with your shoulders. In this posture, extend your legs in the opposite direction, one leg at a time, so as to attain a plank like a posture, which concentrates mainly on your abdominal region. Ensure that your body is straight and even by not allowing your hips to drag down or by not elevating your butt to a greater height. When you pressurize the region around your lower abs muscles, try to replicate the feeling you get when you tighten a seat belt around your waist.

Next, you might want the palms of your hands to rest firmly on the mat, and your heels applying a similar pressure on the mat from the back. Hold this posture for 1–2 minutes and do more if you can. After that, finally return to the original position of rest.

3 complete and thorough reps for this exercise are recommended.

Body-weight squat

This is an advanced squat exercise. You'll have to stand with your feet apart at a distance of your hips. Bend your knees at a small angle and cross your hands over your chest. After attaining this posture, squat and press your entire weight downwards to your feet. Ensure that your feet are pointed and straight, and your knees are parallel to your toes. Tuck your bum in and hold this position. Then retain your original standing position.

It is recommended you do at least 5 sets of this exercise wherein each set comprises of 5 reps.

Swan dive

For this exercise, you'll have to lie down on your stomach with your face towards the floor. Then extend your arms over your head simultaneously keep your toes pointed and elevate the extended arms and legs to a height of 6 inches off ground level. Hold this posture for one count.

After this, you have to rotate your arms out from the sides for a 360-degree rotation. While doing this, exhale deeply and use your arms to touch the tip of your toes with your palms facing downwards to the floor. Hold this posture for one count and return to the original position by bringing your arms back and relax your body.

Repeat this exercise for around 6–8 times every day.

Windshield wiper

In this exercise, you'll have to lie down on your back with your face towards the ceiling while bending your knees to form a 90-degree angle. Extend your arms such that they are parallel to the ground, and stretch your fingers elongating your fingertips. By application of a firm force, press the back of your shoulders on a mat while gracefully moving them away from your ears. Concentrate on the muscles in your waist region, inhale deeply and gradually move your knees to the right. Hold this posture for one second, exhale heavily and retain your initial posture. Repeat the same exercise, but switch to your left leg in order to complete 1 rep.

It is recommended you do a minimum of 5–8 reps every day.

Plank on the ball

You will need a balancing ball to complete this exercise. It is also known as a stability ball in a few markets. Firstly, kneel down on all fours in front of a stability ball while carefully pressing your abdominal region and your hips over the ball's surface. Keep your hands on the floor for maintaining balance and use them for crawling until the ball rolls under your thighs.

Once your body is relatively straight with a slight curve at your back and you have attained a position of balance, hold the posture for approximately 30 seconds. While still, apply pressure so as to achieve adequate elevation for lifting belly button and for tightening your thighs.

Jumping jack reach

In a sitting position, hold your stability ball and jump twice, once with your legs apart and then once when they're together. Repeat this alternate sequence of apart, together, and apart again. After this, stand erect and touch your right hand with the right. Ensure that your right hand is still to balance the ball. Return to your original position with your legs together, and repeat the whole exercise on the other side, completing one rep. 7 reps of this exercise every day is recommended. It is recommended you split the 7 reps into 4 and 3. Complete 4 reps initially and then as an intermediate exercise, do a one-minute Basic Bounce, after which you can continue and complete the remaining 3 reps.

Standing side crunch

For this exercise, you'll have to stand up straight while holding the ball over your head with your elbows bent and parallel to the ground. Ensure that your feet are apart at the distance of your shoulders. Lift your right knee and push it towards one side so as to bring it together with an extended right elbow of yours. You should then retain your starting position and repeat the procedure for your other side. As an intermediate exercise, bounce the ball for 1 minute and then continue the exercise for another 3 repetitions of the sequence.

Basic pump

This exercise is ideal for development of your abdominal region. The exercise for the ease of practice is divided into two steps. In step 1, you'll have to stand with a leg forward and a hoop held around your waist. In this posture, bend your knees at a slight angle and by using the force of your core; spin the hoop around for several rotations just through a unidirectional push. This only happens when the hoop is properly leveled.

In the next step, transfer your weight in order to balance it on your legs, both forward and backward so as to assist in the movement of your hips in forward and backward directions. Apart from moving around, pushing and pulling are used for maintenance of the spin of your hoop.

Circling the sky

This exercise routine is famous among most trainees as it has multiple benefits for various regions of your body, for example, your core, inner thigh, outer hip and butt region. You'll have to lie down with your face towards the ceiling and your hands behind your head. After attaining this posture, tighten the area around your abdominal region, while trying to elevate your upper body to a slight extent. Then, lift your right leg for approximately 5 inches off the ground if possible. If not, you can directly use your left legs by pointing them upwards to the sky.

In the next step, you have to ensure that your core region and your hips are tightened and firm. After this, you will have to race 4 balls (similar to the size of softballs) entirely with your left leg in a clockwise orientation; and then reverse it by circling 4 times in the counterclockwise orientation.

Repeat the entire sequence by lowering your legs and switching to the other side.

Side inclines with a twist

This exercise is ideal for the development of your core, waist, triceps, and biceps and tightening the muscles in those regions.

For this exercise, lie down with your face parallel to the ground on your right side. Place your forearm under a 90-degree angle with your shoulder while keeping your hand perpendicular to your body. Ensure that your legs are stacked for the course of this exercise. Tighten the region around your abs and the right-hand side of your waist. Lift your hips in a manner such that your body from the head to feet is all aligned to form a straight line.

Next, stretch your left arm towards the ceiling while consistently staying applying a threshold pressure on your core region. After that, curve your left arm near the chest region trying to reach for the space between your chest and the ground. Make sure that only the waist is twisting.

Repeat this for 4 times on both sides and follow the sequence 'up, rep, down'.

Brian Adams

Chapter 11: Cyclical Ketogenic Diet

The previous chapters dealt with the importance of ketogenic diet and the role played by it in improving your health. The ketogenic diet, however, has plenty of variations, which were the products of experimentation. One among the variations is the cyclical ketogenic diet. Instead of consuming a significantly lower concentration of carbohydrates during your workout sessions than you do on a general basis, the CKD focuses heavily on one to two days of comprehensive and comparatively higher consumption of carbohydrates so as to refill your muscle glycogen storage bodies. As it requires a person to commit to it entirely, CKDs are not recommended for beginners who aren't able to comply with the intensity of training. For a successful CKD, you must exhaust your entire stored glycogen every week.

CKD is an effective diet for enhanced muscle growth and development. However, with this advantage there is also a disadvantage i.e. you might end up with an elevated level of body fat. Generally with beginners, over consumption of fats is extremely easy, moreover as you exhaust your stored glycogen through physical activity is also profitable at all times. Hence, the diet is not recommended for beginners. Alternatively, beginners can commit themselves entirely to a Targeted Ketogenic Diet, which is another variation of the Standard Ketogenic Diet.

Enhancing Performance with CKD

A cyclical ketogenic diet generally proceeds along the lines of a 6-day commitment to ketogenic dieting and then 1 day of high carb consumption. Apart from a 1-week cycle, many people have experimented with 2-week cycles, wherein 10 days are solely ketogenic and the remaining 4 involve loading heavily on cars. The 2-week split also showed positive results, but it wasn't flexible with respect to the schedule.

The main goal is to switch out from the ketosis temporarily and refill the muscle glycogen, so that you sustain the training performance for your next workout cycle.

The CKD is also not recommended for people who were prescribed to follow the ketogenic diet for combating health related problems like hypertension. Not only is the CKD ineffective for such a crowd, but also could do more harm than heal as certain hormonal reactions which weren't triggered on a low carb diet could show up again and cause disorder to your body's normal functioning.

As the main principle that the CKD follows is complete exhaustion of muscle glycogen, care has been taken for ideal and significant results. For this, a well-defined workout example has to be practiced. The hours of dedication required for training in order to exhaust your glycogen levels completely depends on the concentration of carbs you consume in your foods during your non-ketogenic high carb phase. In terms of the exercise, 2-3 sets of low rep and physically challenging activities, which incorporate heavy weights, are recommended. Similarly, 5-6 sets of high rep and user-friendly exercises, which incorporate moderate weights, are recommended.

Low-Carb Phase

The low-carb phase of the cyclical ketogenic diet follows a similar pattern as that of the Standard Ketogenic Diet (SKD). Your diet should be mainly oriented around these guidelines:

- 18 calories for every pound of your body weight to gain weight.

- 12 calories for every pound of your body weight for efficient weight loss.

- 15-16 calories for every pound of your body weight for effective maintenance of health.

- 30 grams or lower carbohydrate concentration in your meals for the day. However, it is recommended you lower it down to a bare minimum. This is because of the characteristic property of ketosis, which you enter faster only when you consume lower amount of carbs. This is of extreme importance as you have only 5-6 days of low-carb phase.

- If you're a beginner to the diet, set your protein intake target to an approximate of 0.9g per lbs. of lean mass or 150g, whatever is higher. After you have adjusted well to the diet and its regulations, you can set it higher at 1.0-1.2g per pound of lean mass.

Allocate the remaining of your caloric requirements for fats.

Carb-Load Phase

For the efficient transition into a state of anabolism, it is recommended you begin your high-carb diet 5 hours before your workout session. It is prescribed you consume nearly 25-50g of them along with the required amount of protein and fats in order to initiate greater production of liver enzymes which are essential for the breakdown.

Around 5 hours prior to the final workout, in order to boost the concentration of your liver glycogen, you'll have to consume foods, which have a combination of glucose and fructose as their key ingredient. A small amount like 25-50g is ideal to begin with as you can add more whenever required.

Generally people eat whatever they feel is right during their carb-loading phase. No matter how risky the idea of eating high levels of food when on a diet is; it still has the ability to offer significant results. However, for those who prefer to have a more scientific and calculated approach, it is recommended you consult a doctor and follow a certain set of guidelines for efficient nutrient intake in the carb-load phase.

The guidelines are all based on experimental results from people who have dedicated themselves to developing the diet.

For the first half of this phase, 70% of your caloric intake should be carbohydrates i.e. 4.5g per pound of lean mass. The remaining 30% should be split evenly into protein and fats. Moreover, foods with a higher glycemic index should be consumed.

For the second half of this phase, 60% of your caloric intake should be carbs whereas 25% of it should be protein and only 15% from fats. This relates to approximately 2.25g of carbs per pound of lean mass. Unlike the first phase, only foods with a lower glycemic index should be consumed.

Ketosis Post carb up

Emptying your entire glycogen inventory located in the liver is an efficient way to generate the process of ketosis. To do so, you'll have to follow certain steps to ensure that the transition is as smooth as possible.

Do not consume anything after 6 pm on the first day. The following day, wake up early and practice heavy, intense weight training exercises while on an empty stomach. After the workout, follow a ketogenic diet with a very low carb intake for the whole day (0-2% carbs). The next day, wake up at your regular time and practice moderate or medium intensity weight training exercises while on an empty stomach. After the workout, return to your usual ketogenic diet and consume around 3-5% of carbs in the entire day.

Your body will adapt to the terms of the ketogenic diet with time. For example, if you practiced the diet for a year, your body will enter a state of ketosis not only faster but also much more efficiently when compared to less experienced individuals. Apart from the time factor, your training also plays a role in determining your results. The harder you train, the easier your transition to ketosis is. This is because of faster glycogen depletion. Resistance and conditioning exercises offer better results when compared to aerobic training. If you make better choices regarding your carb-foods (for example lower glycemic

Brian Adams

index foods), re-entering the state of ketosis shouldn't be much of a problem for you.

If you are true to your CKD and follow the terms without any deviation or cheating, your body will adapt to the diet faster thereby reducing any risks.

Chapter 12: Breakfast Recipes:

In this chapter, I will give you easy Low carb Ketogenic Breakfast recipes to try out and incorporate in your diet.

<u>Raspberry shake</u>

Ingredients:
- 1 and ½ cup of unsweetened almond milk
- 3 tbsp of cream
- 2 tbsp of Vanilla Whey protein powder
- ½ cup of fresh raspberries

Method:
1. Pour the almond milk into the blender along with the cream.
2. Add the protein powder and raspberries.
3. Blend all the ingredients into a nutritious smoothie.

Brian Adams

Keto-omelet

Ingredients:

- 2 tbsp of unsweetened almond milk
- 4 egg whites
- 1 egg yolk
- ½ cup of spinach
- 1 small onion
- 1 small tomato
- ½ tsp of basil
- Olive oil

Method:

1. First chop the onion, tomato and spinach finely.
2. In another bowl, whisk the egg whites and single yolk with the almond milk. It should become smooth and frothy.
3. Mix the vegetables and egg mixture with some basil.
4. Pour some olive oil into a skillet and let it heat.
5. Then cook your healthy omelet!

Diet bread

Ingredients:

- 250 ml of unsweetened coconut milk
- 3 tbsp of butter
- 1 ½ cup of almond flour
- 2 tsp of baking powder
- 1 tsp of Celtic sea salt
- 3 tbsp of oat fiber
- 5 tbsp of psyllium husk powder
- 1 egg
- 1 cup of hot water

Method:

1. In a bowl, mix the almond flour with the husk powder, salt and baking powder into an even mixture.
2. Over low heat place the solids of the chilled coconut milk and butter. Then remove from heat and whisk well. Whisk in the egg to this.
3. Mix the dry mixture to the wet mixture. Beat it into firm dough. Break this into small parts.
4. Boil the water and pour it into the bowl of dough. Stir it well.
5. Now scoop out your dough and place on the baking sheets. Keep each ball a little apart.
6. Let the bread bake in the oven for about 45 minutes and then let it cool before serving.

Brian Adams

<u>Egg and bacon</u>

Ingredients

- 3 Large Eggs, beaten
- 1/3 Cup full fat Cream
- 1 tablespoon butter
- 4 Slices Bacon
- Slat to taste
- Pepper to taste
- Tomato circles to serve

Method

1. Preheat the oven to 350 Fahrenheit
2. Place the bacon on the baking tray such that they are not overlapping and have enough space.
3. Place them in the oven for 15 to 20 minutes or until completely crispy.
4. Meanwhile, place the eggs in a bowl and beat it.
5. Add in the cream, salt and pepper and beat until well combined.
6. Add the butter to a pan and once it heats, add in the eggs and allow it to scramble.
7. Place the bacon strips on the side of the plate and place the eggs on another corner.
8. Add in the tomato slices and serve hot!

Cajun Cauliflower Hash:

Ingredients:

- 4 tablespoons olive oil or ghee
- 1 onion, chopped into 1/4 inch pieces
- 4 tablespoons garlic, minced
- 2 pounds frozen cauliflower, steamed, chopped into small, squeezed of all moisture
- 2 teaspoons Cajun seasoning
- 16 ounce shaved red pastrami, chopped into 1 inch slices
- 1 green pepper, chopped into 1/4 inch pieces
- A few eggs, fried sunny side up

Method:

1. Place a skillet over medium heat. Add oil. When the oil is heated, add onions. Sauté until the onions are translucent.
2. Add garlic and sauté for a couple of minutes until the garlic is fragrant.
3. Add cauliflower and sauté until it starts getting brown.
4. Add Cajun seasoning. Stir well.
5. Add pastrami and green pepper. Cook until thoroughly heated.
6. Transfer into individual serving bowls.
7. Top with eggs. Sprinkle some more Cajun seasoning over it.

Crunchy Cereal Mix:

Ingredients:

- 4 cups flaked coconut
- 2 teaspoons ground cinnamon
- Stevia to taste (optional)
- Unsweetened milk of your choice
- Low carb fruits of your choice, chopped
- Nuts of your choice

Method:

1. Line a cookie sheet with parchment paper. Spread the coconut flakes over the cookie sheet.
2. Roast in the oven for about 5 minutes. Keep a watch over the oven. Mix the flakes in between a couple of times and roast until light brown.
3. Remove from the oven. Leave it aside to cool. Sprinkle cinnamon powder. It will turn out crunchy in a while.
4. Serve with milk, stevia and fruits and nuts.
5. In case you want to store it, transfer the cooled coconut flakes into an airtight container. Add nuts. Mix well and store it in a cool dry place.

Cream Cheese Pumpkin Pancake:

Ingredients:

For the pumpkin butter:

- 1 tablespoon 100% pumpkin
- 6 tablespoons butter, unsalted
- 1/8 teaspoon stevia

For the pancakes:

- 4 ounces cream cheese
- 4 eggs
- 4 tablespoons coconut flour
- 1/2 tablespoon pumpkin pie spice blend
- 4 tablespoons butter

Method:

1. To make the pumpkin butter: Place butter and pumpkin in a microwavable dish. Mix well. Microwave for 10 seconds on high. Mix well. If not smooth, microwave again for 10 seconds.
2. When the pumpkin butter is smooth, add stevia.
3. To make the pancakes: Add cream cheese, eggs, coconut flour and pumpkin pie spice to the blender. Blend until smooth. Transfer into a bowl.
4. Place a nonstick pan over medium heat. Add 1-tablespoon butter.
5. When the butter melts and begins to brown, pour about 1/4 of the batter. Swirl the pan a bit so that the pancake spreads.

6. Cook until the bottom side is golden brown. Flip sides and cook the other side too.
7. Repeat steps 5 and 6 with the remaining batter.
8. Place a little of the pumpkin butter on the pancake and serve.

Skillet Baked Eggs:

Ingredients:

- 1 cup plain Greek yogurt
- 2 cloves garlic, halved
- Kosher salt to taste
- 3 tablespoons unsalted butter, divided
- 3 tablespoons olive oil
- 5 tablespoons leek, chopped, white and pale green part only
- 3 tablespoons scallions, chopped, white and pale green parts only
- 15 ounces fresh spinach, rinsed
- 2 teaspoons fresh lemon juice
- 6 large eggs
- 1/2 teaspoon crushed red pepper flakes
- 1/4 teaspoon paprika
- 2 teaspoons fresh oregano, chopped

Method:

1. To a small bowl, add yogurt, garlic and a pinch of salt. Mix well and keep aside.
2. Place a skillet over medium heat. Add butter. When the butter is heated, add leeks and scallion.
3. Lower the heat. Cook until softened.
4. Add spinach, salt and lemon juice.
5. Raise the heat to medium high. Sauté for a few minutes until the spinach is wilted.

6. Transfer the contents to a large ovenproof dish. Do not add the excess liquid, which is present in the spinach mixture.
7. Make 6 wells in the mixture.
8. Gently break an egg into each of the wells.
9. Place the dish in a preheated oven. Bake at 300 degree F until the eggs are set.
10. Place a small saucepan over medium low heat. Add the remaining butter. When the butter melts, add the yogurt mixture and a pinch of salt. Cook for a few seconds and add oregano. Cook for 20-30 seconds. Discard the garlic halves.
11. Pour the yogurt mixture over the eggs and serve.

Breakfast Sausages:

Ingredients:

- 1 large green bell pepper, chopped into 1 inch pieces
- 1 large red bell pepper, chopped, chopped into 1 inch pieces
- 1 large yellow bell pepper, chopped, chopped into 1 inch pieces
- 1 large orange bell pepper, chopped, chopped into 1 inch pieces
- 3 teaspoons olive oil
- Spike seasoning to taste or any other seasoning of your choice
- Freshly ground black pepper to taste
- 20 ounces turkey breakfast sausage links
- 1 cup low fat mozzarella, grated

Method:

1. Place the peppers in a greased baking dish. Add 2 teaspoons of oil over the peppers. Mix well.
2. Sprinkle spike seasoning and pepper powder.
3. Bake in a preheated oven at 450 degree F for about 20 minutes.
4. Meanwhile, place a nonstick pan over medium heat. Add the remaining oil. When the oil is heated, add the sausages and cook until well browned all over.

5. Remove and place on your cutting board. When cool enough to handle, chop the sausages into about 2 inch pieces.
6. Add the sausages to the baking dish and bake along with the peppers for about 5-7 minutes.
7. Remove from the oven. Sprinkle cheese over it. Place it back in the oven.
8. Broil for a couple of minutes until the cheese is melted. Serve immediately.

Celery Root Hash Browns:

Ingredients:

- 3-4 celery roots, peeled, grated
- 2 tablespoons coconut oil or ghee
- Salt to taste
- Pepper to taste
- Tomato salsa to serve

Method:

1. Mix salt and pepper to the celery root.
2. Place a pan over medium high heat. Add oil. When the oil is heated, add the grated celery root. Spread it all over the pan to make one large one or else make smaller sized ones. Smaller sized ones can be made in batches.
3. When the bottom side is cooked and golden brown, flip sides and cook the other side too.
4. Chop into wedges.
5. Serve with tomato salsa and scrambled eggs.

Scrambled Tofu:

Ingredients:

- 2 tablespoons olive oil
- 2 bunches green onions, chopped
- 2 cans (14.5 ounce each) peeled, diced tomatoes along with the juice
- 2 packages (12 ounce each) firm silken tofu, drained, mashed
- 1/2 teaspoon ground turmeric
- Salt to taste
- Pepper powder to taste
- 1/2 teaspoon red chili flakes
- 1 cup cheddar cheese, shredded (optional)

Method

1. Place a skillet over medium heat. Add oil. When the oil is heated, add green onions. Sauté until the green onions are tender.
2. Add turmeric, salt and pepper. Sauté for a couple of minutes.
3. Add tofu and tomatoes along with the juice. Mix well.
4. Lower heat and let it heat thoroughly. Sprinkle cheddar cheese if using, and serve.

Spaghetti squash

Ingredients:

- 1 large spaghetti squash
- 6 tbsp of butter
- 1 cup of baked ham
- 1 ½ cup of cream
- 2 egg yolks
- 1 ½ cup of grated cheese
- 1 tsp of garlic paste
- Salt

Method:

1. Cut the squash up and remove the pulp as well as the seeds from the inside.
2. Bake the squash at about 320 degrees and then let it cool.
3. Cut out the strands using a fork.
4. Place a saucepan over medium heat. Melt the butter on this.
5. Sauté the chopped ham on the butter for a couple of minutes.
6. Whisk the egg yolk with the cream and add to the pan.
7. Stir in the garlic and cheese. Let this all cook for a few minutes.
8. Then add the squash and mix well till you get a creamy consistency.
9. Serve hot.

Brian Adams

Chapter 13: Salad Recipes

In this chapter, I have shared some easy Low carb Ketogenic salad recipes that you can try out and maintain good health

<u>Chicken curry salad</u>

Ingredients:

- 1 cup of cooked chicken
- 1/3 cup of celery
- A handful of almonds
- 1 tbsp of butter
- 1 egg yolk
- 1 tbsp of mayonnaise
- 1 tsp of lemon juice
- A sprinkle of salt
- 1 tsp of curry powder

Method:

1. Place a skillet over low heat and melt the butter. Then remove it from heat.
2. Whisk the butter with the egg yolk and then add the mayonnaise. Whisk well.
3. Add the lemon juice, curry powder and salt and whisk it all together. Keep this as your salad dressing.
4. Mix the dressing with the diced chicken. Add some celery and sliced almonds. Your salad is ready!

Egg salad

Ingredients:

- 6 eggs
- 1/3 cup of mayonnaise
- 1 tbsp of butter
- Pinch of ground mustard
- 2 tbsp of minced onion
- Sprinkle of black pepper
- Pinch of salt

Method:

1. First cook the eggs in a pot of boiling water for about 10 minutes.
2. Put the eggs into cold water and let it cool.
3. Then peel and chop the cooked eggs.
4. Mix the eggs with the mayonnaise, butter, mustard, and onion.
5. Add the salt and pepper to taste.
6. It can be kept in the fridge till you want to serve!

Brian Adams

Tofu salad

Ingredients:

- 200 gms firm tofu
- 2 tbsp of soy sauce
- 1 tsp of sesame oil
- 1 tbsp of water
- 1 tsp of minced garlic
- 1 tsp of rice vinegar
- 1 tbsp of lemon juice
- 200 gms of Chinese cabbage
- 1 tbsp of cilantro
- 2 tbsp of virgin coconut oil
- 1 tbsp of peanut butter
- 5 drops of liquid stevia

Method:

1. First press and dry out your tofu.
2. In a bowl mix 1 tsp sesame oil and soy sauce with the vinegar and garlic. Add 1 tsp of lemon juice. This is your marinade.
3. Pour the marinade along with the tofu into a Ziploc bag and leave it for an hour.
4. Then bake the chopped tofu for about 30 minutes at 325 degrees or so.
5. While the tofu is baking, make the rest of your salad.
6. Chop up the cilantro and mix with the remaining ingredients except the Chinese cabbage and lime juice.

7. Slice up the Chinese cabbage.
8. Just before adding the tofu, mix the sliced cabbage and lemon juice into the dressing.
9. Then add the tofu and mix.

Sirloin Steak Salad with Gorgonzola and Pine Nuts

Ingredients:

- 1 sirloin steak of about a pound and an inch thick
- 2 1/2 tablespoons olive oil
- Kosher salt to taste
- Freshly ground black pepper to taste
- 1 teaspoon fresh rosemary
- 1/2 tablespoon red wine vinegar
- 1 teaspoon Dijon mustard or to taste
- 1 clove garlic, minced
- 4 cups mixed baby greens
- 2 tablespoons pine nuts, toasted
- 3 ounce Gorgonzola cheese, crumbled

Method:

1. Apply the steak with 1/2-tablespoon olive oil. Rub well. Season with salt and pepper.
2. Take a little of the rosemary and rub it over the steak. Leave aside for an hour at room temperature or refrigerate for at least 4 hours, uncovered.
3. If you refrigerate it, then remove from the oven about 45 minutes before you grill it.
4. Prepare a grill, either a charcoal grill or gas grill or a grill pan placed over high heat.
5. Place the steak on the grill rack of whatever method you are using to grill. Grill for a couple of minutes. Flip sides and grill the other side for a couple of minutes or until done.

6. Transfer on to a plate. Cover it loosely for a few minutes. When cool enough to handle, cut the steak across the grains.

7. Meanwhile, add vinegar, mustard, garlic, salt and pepper to a bowl. Whisk constantly. Whisking constantly, pour the remaining oil in a thin stream. Continue whisking until the mixture is emulsified.

8. To serve: Place the greens in a serving bowl. Place the steak slices over it. Sprinkle pine nuts and Gorgonzola cheese. Sprinkle the dressing and serve immediately.

Caper and Lemon Salad:

Ingredients:

- 3 pounds salmon fillet
- Salt to taste
- Pepper to taste
- Juice of a lemon or to taste
- 1 teaspoon lemon zest, grated
- 1/3 cup canned capers, drained, rinsed
- 3 stalks celery, chopped
- 3 teaspoon fresh dill, chopped
- 3 tablespoons extra virgin olive oil

Method:

1. Season the salmon with salt and pepper and bake in a preheated oven at 350 degree F for 10 minutes or until the salmon is flaky.
2. Transfer the salmon to a serving bowl. Add lemon juice, lemon zest, capers, celery, dill and olive oil and toss.
3. Place in the refrigerator until use.

Caesar Salad:

Ingredients:

- 8 anchovy filets
- 4 garlic cloves
- 1/2 cup parmesan, grated
- 24 whole leaves of romaine hearts, rinsed, pat dried
- 4 ounces pork rinds, chopped in small pieces
- 1/2 cup parmesan cheese, shaved for garnish
- 1/2 cup homemade mayonnaise - refer chapter 4

Method:

1. Add anchovies, garlic and Parmesan.
2. Blend again on low until the mixture is well combined and of smooth texture.
3. Lay the lettuce leaves on individual plates. Spread a little of the mayonnaise over the leaves.
4. Divide the pork pieces amongst the plates.
5. Serve garnished with Parmesan.

Keto Cobb Salad:

Ingredients:

For the dressing:

- 2 tablespoons olive oil
- 2 tablespoons apple cider vinegar
- 2 teaspoons lemon juice
- 2 teaspoons Dijon mustard
- 1 clove garlic, minced
- Salt to taste
- Pepper powder to taste

For the salad:

- Cooking spray
- 1 cup ham, chopped into cubes
- 8 cherry tomatoes
- 1/4 cup blue cheese, shredded
- 4 hard boiled eggs, sliced
- 4 cups romaine lettuce chopped
- 1 avocado, peeled, pitted, diced
- 4 slices turkey bacon

Method:

1. Mix together all the ingredients of the dressing. Whisk well and keep aside.

2. Place a pan over medium heat. Spray with cooking spray. Add the ham and cook for about 5 minutes. Remove from heat and keep aside.
3. Place the lettuce at the bottom of a large salad bowl.
4. Lay the tomatoes, avocado, blue cheese, ham, eggs and ban in rows.
5. Sprinkle the dressing and serve.

Egg Salad 2

Ingredients:

- 9 eggs, hard boiled, chopped into small pieces
- 3 tablespoons mayonnaise
- 1 1/2 teaspoon Dijon mustard
- 1 1/2 teaspoon lemon juice
- Salt to taste
- Pepper to taste
- Lettuce leaves to serve

Method:

1. Mix together the eggs, mayonnaise, mustard, lemon juice, salt and pepper in a bowl.
2. Adjust the seasonings if necessary.
3. Serve over lettuce leaves.

Spinach and Apple Salad

Ingredients:

For the salad:

- 8 cups baby spinach leaves, rinsed
- 1 cup red onion, thinly sliced
- 1/2 cup blue cheese, crumbled
- 1 apple, cored, cut into small cubes

For the dressing:

- 1 cup cold pressed olive oil
- 2/3 cup red wine vinegar
- 2 cloves garlic, minced
- 1/2 cup feta cheese, crumbled
- 8 slices thin bacon, cooked, crumbled to serve

Method:

1. To make the dressing: Blend together all the ingredients of the dressing until smooth. Transfer into a glass bowl. Add bacon and mix well.
2. Place the spinach leaves over a large serving platter. Lay the apple pieces over the spinach.
3. Drizzle the dressing all over the salad. Toss and serve.

Greek Cucumber Salad:

Ingredients:

- 2 tablespoons red wine vinegar
- 2 tablespoons extra virgin olive oil
- 2 tablespoons finely chopped fresh oregano,
- 2 teaspoons Dijon mustard
- Salt to taste
- Freshly ground black pepper to taste
- 8 cups cucumbers, peeled, chopped
- 2 cups cherry tomatoes, halved
- 1 cup mixed olives, pitted
- 1 red onion, thinly sliced
- 1/4 cup feta cheese, crumbled
- 1/4 cup fresh basil, chopped

Method:

1. Whisk together in a large bowl, oil, vinegar, oregano, mustard, salt and pepper.
2. Add rest of the ingredients. Toss well and serve.

Salmon and chickpeas salad:

Ingredients:

- 1 can chickpeas, rinsed, drained
- 3 stalks celery, thinly sliced
- 2 shallots, finely minced
- 2 cloves of garlic, finely minced
- 1 bell pepper, thinly sliced
- 1 medium cucumber, halved, sliced
- 1/2 pint tomatoes, halved
- 1/4 olive oil or to taste
- Juice of 1/2 a lemon
- Zest of 1/2 a lemon
- 1 tablespoon red wine vinegar
- 1/2 teaspoon kosher salt or to taste
- 1/2 teaspoon fresh or dried dill
- 1/4 teaspoon freshly ground black pepper
- 1/4 teaspoon smoked paprika
- 1/4 teaspoon ground cumin
- 1/4 teaspoon crushed red pepper flakes
- 2 cans salmon, drained

Method:

1. Add all the ingredients to a large bowl. Toss well and refrigerate for an hour.
2. Taste and adjust the seasoning if necessary and serve.

Brian Adams

Chapter 14: Soups Recipes

In this chapter, I have shared some delicious Low carb Ketogenic soup recipes. These are great as a snack for the untimely hunger pangs.

Chicken broth

Ingredients:

- ½ kg of organic chicken
- 1 tsp of salt
- 1 small onion
- Celery
- 1 carrot
- 1 garlic clove
- 1 ½ quart of water
- Dried thyme leaves
- Parsley
- 3 peppercorns

Brian Adams

Method:

1. Keep your oven preheated to 375 degrees.
2. Mix the chicken with the cut up onion, celery, and garlic. Sprinkle salt over this. Roast for about an hour.
3. When the chicken is roasted, transfer it all into a stockpot.
4. Put on medium heat.
5. Add the water to the pot. Stir in the thyme, parsley and peppercorns.
6. Let the pot simmer over low heat for 3 hours. Gently skim off anything off the top.
7. Then let the pot cool for about an hour and then strain.
8. It can be stored in the freezer.

Quick Tomato Soup:

Ingredients:

- 8 roma tomatoes
- 1 cup sun dried tomatoes
- 1 cup raw macadamia nuts
- 2 teaspoons sea salt
- 1/2 cup fresh basil
- 1 teaspoon white pepper powder or to taste
- 1/2 teaspoon black pepper powder or to taste
- 2 cloves garlic
- 8 cups hot water

Method:

1. Add all the ingredients to your food processor and blend until smooth.
2. Heat it thoroughly.
3. Ladle into individual soup bowls and serve hot.

Cream of Mushroom Soup:

Ingredients:

- 3 cups cauliflower florets
- 2 cups unsweetened original almond milk
- 1 1/2 teaspoons onion powder
- 1/2 teaspoon Himalayan rock salt
- Freshly ground pepper, to taste
- 1 teaspoon extra-virgin olive oil
- 2 1/2 cups white mushrooms, diced
- 1 yellow onion, diced

Method:

1. Add cauliflower, milk, onion powder, salt and pepper to a saucepan.
2. Place the pan over medium heat. Bring to a boil.
3. Lower heat and simmer until the cauliflowers are soft. Puree the cauliflower using an immersion blender.
4. Meanwhile, place a saucepan over medium heat. Add oil. When the oil is heated, add onions and sauté for a couple of minutes. Add mushrooms and sauté until the onions are light brown.
5. Add the cauliflower puree. Mix well and bring to a boil.
6. Reduce heat and simmer for 10-12 minutes.
7. Ladle into individual soup bowls and serve hot.

Bacon Cheeseburger Soup:

Ingredients:

- 10 slices bacon
- 24 ounce ground beef
- 4 tablespoons butter
- 6 cups beef broth
- 1 teaspoon garlic powder
- 1 teaspoon onion powder
- 4 teaspoons brown mustard
- Kosher salt to taste
- Black pepper powder to taste
- 1 teaspoon red pepper flakes
- 2 teaspoons ground cumin
- 2 teaspoons chili powder or to taste
- 5 tablespoons tomato paste
- 2 medium dill pickle, diced
- 2 cups cheddar cheese, shredded
- 6 ounce cream cheese
- 1 cup heavy cream

Method:

1. Place a skillet over medium heat. Add bacon and cook until crisp. Remove and keep aside on a plate.
2. To the same skillet, add beef. Cook until the bottom side is brown. Flip sides and cook the other side too.
3. Transfer the beef to a large pot. Place the pot over medium heat. Add butter, cumin, salt, pepper, red chili flakes, onion powder, garlic powder, brown mustard and chili powder. Mix well.

4. Pour the beef broth and mix well.
5. Add tomato paste, cheese and pickle. Mix well and bring to a boil.
6. Lower heat, cover and simmer for about 30 minutes.
7. Remove from heat. Crumble the cooked bacon and add to the soup. Mix well.
8. Ladle into individual soup bowls and serve hot.

Chicken Enchilada Soup:

Ingredients:

- 6 tablespoons olive oil
- 6 stalks celery, diced
- 2 medium red bell pepper, diced
- 4 teaspoons garlic, minced
- 8 cups chicken broth
- 2 cups tomatoes, diced
- 2 cups cream cheese
- 12 ounces chicken, cooked, shredded
- 1 1/2 tablespoons ground cumin
- 2 teaspoons oregano
- 2 teaspoons chili powder
- 1 teaspoon cayenne pepper
- 1 cup cilantro, chopped
- Juice of a lime

Method:

1. Place a large pot over medium heat. Add oil. When the oil is heated, add celery and pepper. Sauté until the celery is softened.
2. Add tomatoes and sauté for a couple of minutes.
3. Add cumin, oregano, chili powder and cayenne pepper. Mix well.
4. Add chicken broth and cilantro. Bring to a boil.
5. Lower heat and simmer for about 20 minutes.

6. Add cream cheese. Mix well and bring to a boil. Simmer again for about 30 minutes.
7. Add lime juice, mix well and garnish with cilantro.
8. Ladle into individual soup bowls and serve hot.

Egg Drop Soup:

Ingredients:

- 4 eggs, beaten
- 8 cups of bone broth or 8 cups of water mixed with 4 bouillon cubes
- A pinch of red pepper flakes or to taste
- Freshly ground pepper to taste
- 1 scallion, chopped

Method:

1. Pour the bone broth or water and bouillon cubes to a large saucepan. Place the saucepan over high heat.
2. Add pepper powder and chili powder and bring to a boil.
3. Gently pour in the beaten eggs and stir constantly until it begins to boil.
4. Garnish with scallions.
5. Ladle into individual soup bowls and serve hot.

Spicy Cauliflower soup:

Ingredients:

- 2 large cauliflower heads, chopped into florets
- 2 medium turnips, peeled, chopped
- 2 small white onions, chopped
- 4 cups vegetable stock
- 2 medium chorizos (optional)
- 1/3 cup ghee or butter
- Salt to taste
- 2 medium spring onions, chopped
- Cheddar cheese, shredded to garnish

Method:

1. Place a large saucepan over medium heat. Add 4 tablespoons ghee. When the ghee is melted, add onions. Sauté until the onions are light brown.
2. Add cauliflower and sauté for a few minutes. Add broth, cover and bring to a boil.
3. Simmer for about 10 minutes.
4. Meanwhile, place a skillet over medium heat. Add the remaining butter. When the butter melts, add turnips and chorizos if you are using. Sauté until the turnips are tender. If you do not prefer turnips, you can add some cauliflower florets instead.
5. Transfer half the turnips and chorizo to the saucepan. Mix well. Blend with an immersion blender.
6. Ladle into individual soup bowls, sprinkle the remaining turnips

7. Sprinkle salt and cayenne pepper. Garnish with cheddar cheese and serve hot.

Brian Adams

Beef and Vegetable Soup:

Ingredients:

- 12 cups beef stock
- 2 medium turnips, peeled, finely chopped
- 1 daikon radish, finely chopped
- 1 baby bok choy, finely chopped
- 1 medium onion, chopped
- 2 cups portabella mushrooms, finely chopped
- 1 cup zucchini, finely chopped
- 1/2 cup crimini mushrooms, finely chopped
- 1 1/4 pounds, beef stew meat, chopped into small pieces
- 1/2 tablespoon oil
- Salt to taste
- Pepper powder to taste

Method:

1. Place a large saucepan over medium heat. Add stock, turnip, radish, and bok choy.
2. Meanwhile place a frying pan over medium heat. Add oil and sauté the onions until brown. Transfer into the saucepan.
3. Add crimini mushrooms to the same frying pan and sauté until brown. Transfer to the saucepan.
4. Add mushrooms to the same frying pan and sauté until brown. Transfer to the saucepan.
5. Add meat to the same frying pan and sauté until brown. Transfer to the saucepan.

6. Bring to a boil. Lower heat, cover and simmer for a couple of hours until the meat is cooked. Season with salt and pepper.
7. Ladle into soup bowls and serve.

Brian Adams

Chapter 15: Accompaniments Recipes

In this chapter, I give you some tasty Low carb Ketogenic accompaniments recipes that will go perfectly well with your mains

Cauliflower soup for Snack

Ingredients

- 1 large Cauliflower
- 2 tablespoons Olive Oil
- 1 large red onion
- 4 Slices Bacon
- 12 ounces Cheddar cheese
- 1 teaspoon rosemary, chopped
- 3 cups vegetable broth
- ¼ cup low fat Cream

- 1 ounce parmesan Cheese
- 1 tablespoons Minced Garlic
- Salt to taste
- Pepper to taste

Method

1. Clean and separate the florets from the cauliflower and place it on an aluminum foil and sprinkle the salt and pepper over it.
2. Place it in a 375 degrees pre heated oven for 35 minutes.
3. In a medium skillet, add in the bacon and allow it's fat to release.
4. Remove the bacon and add the chopped onion to the bacon fat and cook until golden.
5. Add in the garlic and the rosemary and cook it for a minute or two minutes.
6. Add in the vegetable broth and the cauliflower and cook it covered for 20 minutes.
7. While it mix simmers, add in the cheese and give it a good mix.
8. You can make use of a hot blender to place in the soup and blend or transfer it to a blender and blend it until creamy.
9. Add in the bacon and whizz until completely smooth.
10. Place it back to the pan and heat for a further 5 minutes and serve hot.

Keto Buns:

Ingredients:

Dry ingredients:

- 3 cups almond flour or almond meal
- 2/3 cup psyllium husk powder (powder the psyllium husk)
- 1 cup coconut flour
- 1 cup flax meal
- 1 1/2 tablespoons garlic powder
- 1 1/2 tablespoons onion powder
- 1 1/2 tablespoons cream of tartar
- 2 teaspoons baking soda
- 2 teaspoons sea salt
- 10 tablespoons seeds of your choice (sunflower or flax or poppy or caraway seeds or sesame)

Wet ingredients:

- 12 large egg whites
- 4 large eggs
- 4 cups boiling water

Method:

1. Mix together all the dry ingredients except the seeds in a bowl.
2. Add the egg whites and eggs and whisk well until thick dough is formed.
3. Add boiling water and mix well.

4. Spoon about 2 tablespoons of the batter for each bun on to a nonstick baking tray lined with parchment paper. Leave a gap between 2 buns.
5. Press the seeds you are using on to the buns.
6. Bake in a preheated oven at 350 degree F for about 45 minutes or until done.
7. Remove the tray from the oven. When it is slightly cooled, transfer on to a wire rack to cool completely.

Keto Bread:

Ingredients:

- 6 large eggs
- 1 cup almond flour
- 3 teaspoons baking powder
- 4 tablespoons butter

Method:

1. Add all the ingredients to a bowl. Whisk well until the batter is smooth and well aerated.
2. Transfer to a greased baking pan.
3. Bake in a preheated oven at 390 degree F for about 20 minutes or until done.
4. If your want to make muffins, then pour the batter into greased muffin tins.

Cheese Garlic Bread:

Ingredients:

- 2 1/2 cups almond flour
- 2 tablespoons coconut flour
- 6 egg whites, beaten until fluffy
- 4 tablespoons olive oil or avocado oil
- 1/2 cup warm water
- 2 teaspoons live yeast granules
- 2 teaspoons coconut sugar
- 1 cup mozzarella cheese, shredded
- 1/2 teaspoon salt
- 4 teaspoons baking powder
- 1/2 teaspoon garlic powder
- 1 teaspoon xanthan or guar gum (optional)

For topping:

- 2 cups mozzarella cheese, shredded
- 4 tablespoons butter, melted
- 1/2 teaspoon garlic powder
- 1/2 teaspoon salt
- 1 teaspoon Italian seasoning

Method:

1. Mix together all the dry ingredients in a bowl.

2. In a small bowl, add warm water and sugar. Mix until dissolved. Add yeast and keep aside for a few minutes.
3. To the dry ingredients, add olive oil and the water mixture. Mix well with a rubber spatula. Add eggs and mix again.
4. Add mozzarella and mix until well combined.
5. Transfer the batter on to a lined or greased baking sheet.
6. Bake at 400 degree F for about 15 minutes or the sides of the bread are turning golden brown. Remove from the oven and keep aside to cool.
7. Sprinkle mozzarella cheese over the bread. Season with Italian seasoning.
8. Bake for a while until the cheese is melted.
9. Remove from the oven and serve.

Homemade Mayonnaise:

Ingredients:

- 2 egg yolks
- 1 cup avocado oil
- 6 tablespoons Apple Cider Vinegar
- 2 teaspoons Dijon mustard

Method:

1. Add yolk, apple cider vinegar, and mustard to a bowl. Blend with an immersion blender.
2. With the blender running on low speed, pour avocado oil in a thin stream. Do not move the blender from the position that it is running. Slowly the mixture will emulsify.
3. Remove from the blender and transfer into a bowl.

Mashed Cauliflower (mock mashed potatoes):

Ingredients:

- 3 heads cauliflower, made into small floret's
- 6 tablespoons heavy cream
- 3 tablespoons butter
- 3/4 cup cheddar cheese, shredded
- Salt to taste
- Pepper to taste

Method:

1. Place the cauliflower florets in a microwave safe bowl along with 1-tablespoon cream and 1 tablespoon butter.
2. Microwave on high for 6 minutes, uncovered. Add the remaining butter and cream.
3. Mix well and microwave on high for 6-7 minutes more.
4. Remove from microwave. Add cheese and blend with an immersion blender until smooth or blend in the food processor.
5. Add salt and pepper to taste.

Zucchini Banana Bread:

Ingredients:

- 1 1/2 cups coconut flour
- 2 1/4 teaspoons baking soda
- 1 1/2 teaspoons salt
- 3 tablespoons ground cinnamon
- 1 teaspoon nutmeg
- 12 eggs
- 2 tablespoons raw honey
- 3 cups zucchini, finely shredded, squeezed of all the moisture
- 3 ripe bananas, peeled, mashed
- 3 tablespoons coconut oil
- 1 1/2 cups walnuts, chopped, (optional)

Method:

1. Mix together eggs, honey, oil, and banana in a bowl.
2. Add shredded zucchini, coconut flour, baking soda, salt, cinnamon and nutmeg. Mix well combined to get a smooth batter. Add walnuts if using.
3. Pour the batter into a greased bread pan or lined with parchment paper (fill it ¾ full).
4. Bake in a preheated oven at 350 degree for about 45 minutes or until done.

Zucchini Pasta / Noodles:

Ingredients:

- 4 zucchini peeled
- 2 tablespoons olive oil
- 6 tablespoons water
- Salt to taste
- Pepper powder to taste

Method:

1. Use a vegetable peeler and peel strips of the zucchini lengthwise. Discard the seed part.
2. Place a nonstick pan over medium heat. Add olive oil.
3. When the oil is hot, add the zucchini. Sauté for a couple of minutes. Add water. Cook for a while until the water dries up. Season with salt and pepper. Serve with sauce of your choice.
4. To make the noodles, peel strands of the zucchini with a julienne peeler or make noodles using a spiralizer.
5. Step 2 remains the same.

Brian Adams

Chapter 16: Snacks Recipes

This chapter has some easy Low carb Ketogenic snack recipes that you can munch on between meals.

Kale chips

Ingredients:

- 4 cups of Kale leaves
- ½ cup of bacon grease
- 3 tbsp of butter
- 2 tsp of kosher salt

Method:

1. Keep your oven preheated to 370 degrees approximately.
2. Remove the stems from the kale leaves and tear it up.
3. Take a pan and heat the butter and bacon grease.
4. Add salt into the pan.

5. Put the kale in a Ziploc bag and add the grease to this. Shake well to mix it all in.
6. Then spread out the leaves onto your baking tray and let it cook for about 20 minutes.
7. The leaves should turn brownish and crispy.

Tortilla chips

Ingredients:

- 3 flaxseed tortillas
- 2 tbsp of absorbed oil
- 2 tbsp of shredded cheese
- 1/3 cup of fresh prepared salsa
- Pinch of salt and pepper

Method:

1. Cut the tortilla chips into desired sizes.
2. Use a deep fryer to fry the chips in the oil till they are brown.
3. Then sprinkle with the salt and pepper.
4. Serve with cheese and salsa.

Brian Adams

Vegetable quiche

Ingredients:

-
    1 cup of sliced vegetables including carrots, peppers and cauliflower.
- 1 small onion
- 2 cups of cheese
- 1 tbsp of butter
- 4 eggs
- 1 cup of cream
- 1 tsp of salt
- A little black pepper

Method:

1. Place a skillet over medium heat and melt the butter.
2. Slice up the onion and add to the butter along with the vegetables.
3. Sauté for a while and then remove from heat.
4. Take your quiche pans and first layer it with some shredded cheese.
5. Add a layer of your sautéed vegetables over the cheese and spread evenly.
6. Whisk the eggs in a bowl with the salt, black pepper and cream till it is frothy. Pour this over the vegetables.
7. Keep the oven preheated before sliding the quiche pans in. It should be done in 20-30 minutes.

8. To check if the quiche is baked, slide the tip of a knife through the center and then pull out. If it comes out clean then you're done!

Smoked Zucchini Chips:

Ingredients:

- 3 medium zucchinis
- Salt to taste
- 2 tablespoons olive oil
- 3 teaspoons smoked paprika
- Pepper powder to taste

Method:

1. Cut the zucchini into 1/4th inch thick slices, crosswise with a slicer or a knife.
2. Place the zucchini on a sieve in layers sprinkled with salt and pepper. Keep aside for an hour. Some moisture content of the zucchini will drain out.
3. Pat dry the zucchini slices with a paper towel and place on a greased baking tray.
4. Brush the top of the slices with oil. Sprinkle paprika and pepper.
5. Bake in a preheated oven at 250 degree F for 45 minutes. Turn of the oven and let the chips remain inside for an hour so that it remains crispy.

Lettuce Wraps:

Ingredients:

- 8 leaves iceberg lettuce
- 4 slices roast turkey
- 1/2 cucumber, sliced
- 250 grams hummus
- 1/4 teaspoon paprika

Method:

1. Spread 4 lettuce leaves on your working area.
2. Place a slice of turkey on 4 of the leaves.
3. Lay a few slices of cucumber. Add a dollop of hummus. Sprinkle paprika.
4. Fold over and wrap another lettuce leaf all over it.

Prosciutto wrapped muffins:

Ingredients:

- 6 tablespoons coconut oil or ghee
- 1 medium onion, finely diced
- 5 cloves garlic, minced
- 3/4 pound crimini mushrooms, thinly sliced
- 3/4 pound frozen spinach, thawed and squeezed dry
- 12 large eggs
- 1/2 cup coconut milk
- 4 tablespoons coconut flour
- 1 1/2 cups cherry tomatoes, halved
- 7.5 ounces of prosciutto
- Kosher salt to taste
- Freshly ground pepper to taste

Method:

1. Place a large skillet over medium heat. Add half the oil. When the oil is melted, add onions and sauté until the onions are translucent.
2. Add garlic and sauté for a couple of minutes until fragrant.
3. Add mushrooms and sauté until almost dry. Add salt and pepper. Remove from heat and keep aside on a plate.
4. In a larger bowl, whisk together coconut milk, coconut flour, salt, and pepper until well combined.
5. Add the mushrooms and spinach and mix well.
6. Grease the muffin tins with the remaining oil.
7. Place a prosciutto inside the muffin cup in such a manner that the bottom as well as the sides are completely covered.

8. Pour the batter into each of the prosciutto cups.
9. Bake in a preheated oven at 375 degree F for about 20 minutes or until set.
10. Remove from the oven and let it cool a little. Remove the muffins and place on a wire rack to cool completely.

Brian Adams

Healthy Granola Bars:

Ingredients:

- 3 cups macadamia nuts
- 3 cups almonds
- 3 cups sunflower seeds
- 3 cups unsweetened flaked coconut
- 3 eggs
- 3/4 cup coconut butter
- 3/4 cup organic peanut butter
- 1 1/2 cups dark chocolate chips
- 3 tablespoons vanilla extract
- 3 teaspoons pumpkin pie spice

Method:

1. Blend together all the ingredients in a blender until smooth. If you like them nutty, then make a coarse paste.
2. Transfer to a greased ovenproof dish. Press well.
3. Bake in a preheated oven at 350 degree F for 15 minutes or golden brown.
4. Cool slightly. Slice into pieces and serve.

Peanut butter Sandwiches:

Ingredients:

- 2 large banana, sliced evenly (say about 30 slices)
- 6 medium strawberries, sliced evenly (say about 15 slices)
- 3 tablespoons peanut butter

Method:

1. Spread 15 banana slices over a plate and spread the peanut butter over it.
2. Lay a slice of strawberry on each of the 15 buttered bananas.
3. Cover each with the remaining 15 slices of banana.
4. Mini peanut butter sandwiches are ready to serve.

Brian Adams

Fish Nuggets:

Ingredients:

- 3 pounds fish like cod or snapper, rinsed, cut into nuggets
- 6 eggs, beaten
- 1 1/2 cup shredded coconut
- Sea salt to taste
- 1 1/2 teaspoon garlic powder
- 1 teaspoon pepper powder or to taste
- 3/4 cup coconut oil

Method:

1. Add coconut, salt, garlic powder and pepper powder to a bowl. Mix well.
2. Dip the nuggets first in the beaten egg and then roll in the coconut mixture and set aside on a plate.
3. Add ¼ cup oil to a skillet and place on medium heat.
4. Add the nuggets in batches and cook until brown.
5. Repeat steps 3 and 4 with the remaining nuggets. Add more oil if required.
6. Serve with any dip of your choice.

Chapter 17: Vegetarian Main Course Recipes

Butter Paneer curry:

Ingredients:

- 2 cups Paneer, chopped into cubes
- ½ cup water
- ½ cup crushed tomatoes
- ¼ cup heavy whipping cream
- 2 tablespoons butter
- ½ tablespoon olive oil
- 1 teaspoon coconut oil
- 1 teaspoon garlic paste
- 1 teaspoon ginger paste
- ½ teaspoon garam masala
- ½ teaspoon coriander powder

- ½ teaspoon pepper powder
- 1 teaspoon salt or to taste
- ¼ teaspoon paprika
- ¼ teaspoon chili powder
- ¼ teaspoon Kashmiri chili powder
- A sprig of cilantro, chopped

Method:

1. Place a pan on medium heat. Add butter and coconut oil.

2. When the butter melts, add ginger and garlic. Sauté for a couple of minutes until fragrant.

3. Add tomatoes, coriander powder, garam masala, paprika, red chili powder, and salt. Mix well and simmer for about 3-5 minutes.

4. Add Paneer and water. Simmer for about 5 minutes. Reduce heat and add cream. Mix well. Bring to a boil.

5. Mix well and simmer for about 4-5 minutes.

6. Garnish with cilantro and serve hot.

Eggplant and Mushrooms with Peanut Sauce

Ingredients:

- 4 Japanese eggplants cut into 1 inch thick round slices
- 3/4 pound shiitake mushrooms, stems discarded, halved
- 3 tablespoons smooth peanut butter
- 2 1/2 tablespoons rice vinegar
- 1 1/2 tablespoons soy sauce
- 1 1/2 tablespoons, peeled, fresh ginger, finely grated
- 1 1/2 tablespoons light brown sugar
- Coarse salt to taste
- 3 scallions, cut into 2 inch lengths, thinly sliced lengthwise

Method:

1. Place the eggplants and mushroom in a steamer. Steam the eggplant and mushrooms until tender. Transfer to a bowl.
2. To a small bowl add peanut butter and vinegar and whisk.
3. Add rest of the ingredients and whisk well. Add this to the bowl of eggplants. Add scallions and mix well.
4. Serve hot.

Brian Adams

Quinoa, Broccoli, and Cheese Casserole:

Ingredients:

- 1 cup quinoa, rinsed in a fine sieve
- 2 cups low sodium vegetable broth/2 cups water with 2 vegetable bouillon cube
- 1 teaspoons salt free seasoning blend or to taste
- 1 1/2 tablespoons extra virgin olive oil
- 2 medium onions, quartered and thinly sliced
- 2 medium broccoli heads, cut into bite sized pieces
- 1/2 cup sliced sun-dried tomatoes or sliced black olives
- Salt to taste
- Freshly ground pepper to taste
- 1 1/2 cup grated cheddar cheese
- 3 medium tomatoes, sliced

Method:

1. Add quinoa, broth and seasoning to a saucepan. Place the saucepan over low heat. Cook until the moisture is absorbed. Remove from heat and keep aside for a while. Fluff with a fork.
2. Place a skillet over medium heat. Add oil. When the oil is heated, add onions. Sauté for 8-10 minutes until golden brown.
3. Add broccoli florets and a little water. Cover and cook until the broccoli is crisp and tender.

4. Transfer the broccoli to a greased casserole dish. Add half the cheddar cheese, dried tomatoes, salt and pepper. Lay the tomato slices over the mixture.
5. Sprinkle the remaining cheese.
6. Bake in a preheated oven at 400 degree F for about 20-30 minutes until the top is golden brown. Cool for 5 minutes and serve.

Brian Adams

Chapter 18: Vegetarian Recipes with Eggs

<u>Courgetti Bolognese:</u>

Ingredients:

- 4 straight courgettes
- 3 eggs
- 1 ½ cups Quorn mince
- 1 large onion, peeled, finely chopped
- 6 cloves garlic, minced
- 3 cans plum tomatoes
- ½ cup parmesan cheese
- 2 teaspoons dried oregano
- Salt to taste
- Pepper powder to taste

Method:

1. Cut the sides of the courgette lengthwise such that it resembles a rectangular block. Now slice the rectangular block into ½ centimeter thick slices.
2. Slice each of the slices into ½ centimeter long strips (on the whole you should have long strips of ½ centimeter thick and ½ centimeter wide).
3. Place the strips in a bowl and season with salt.
4. Meanwhile, whisk together eggs, salt, pepper and ½ teaspoon oregano. Pour this mixture over the courgette strips and keep it aside for a while.
5. To make sauce: Place a large pan over medium heat. Add oil. When the oil is heated, add onions, garlic and remaining oregano and sauté until the onions are translucent.
6. Add mushrooms, Stir well. Cover and cook for about 5 minutes.
7. Reduce heat to low. Add tomatoes, mix well, cover and simmer for around 10 minutes.
8. Add Quorn mince salt and pepper. Mix well. Cover and simmer for another 15-20 minutes.
9. Meanwhile place a large pan over medium heat. Add oil and the courgettes. Sauté for about 10 minutes or until the courgettes are softened.
10. To serve: Place some Courgetti over individual serving plates. Pour the sauce over the Courgetti and serve,

Zucchini Casserole:

Ingredients:

- 12 cups zucchini, diced
- 1 red bell pepper chopped
- 1 yellow bell pepper, chopped
- 1 cup quinoa, cook according to the package instructions
- 1 ½ cups cheddar cheese, shredded
- ¾ cup olive oil
- 1 ½ teaspoons dried basil
- 3 eggs, beaten
- Salt to taste
- Pepper powder to taste

Method:

1. Mix together all the ingredients in a bowl. Transfer to a greased baking dish.
2. Spread all over.
3. Bake in a preheated oven at 350 degree F until top is golden brown.

Brian Adams

Spinach Muenster Quiche:

Ingredients:

- 12 ounces muenster cheese, sliced
- 30 ounce frozen spinach, thawed, drained, squeezed of extra moisture
- 3 eggs
- ½ cup parmesan cheese, grated
- 16 ounces cream cheese, softened
- Salt to taste
- Pepper powder to taste
- 2 teaspoons garlic powder
- 8 ounces muenster cheese, sliced, for topping

Method:

1. Place 12 ounces Muenster cheese slices all over a large pie pan.
2. Mix together eggs, Parmesan, cream cheese, salt, pepper and garlic powder. Transfer into the pie pan over the cheese slices. Spread it well.
3. Place the remaining 8 ounce slices over it.
4. Bake in a preheated oven at 350 degree F for about 30 minutes or golden brown and serve.

Chapter 19: Chicken Main Course Recipes

Chicken curry

Ingredients:

- 3 chicken drumsticks
- 1 tbsp of coconut oil
- 1 green chili
- 1 garlic clove
- 1 tsp of turmeric powder
- 1/3 cup of coconut milk
- 1/3 cup of water
- Pinch of salt
- 1 lemongrass stalk
- 1 tsp of chopped cilantro
- 1 shallot
- ½ tsp of ginger paste

Method:

1. Make a paste out of the ginger, garlic, green chili and shallot. This can be done using a blender or just mashed using a pestle.
2. Place a pan over medium heat and add the coconut oil.
3. Stir in the paste you just made and let it sauté.
4. After a couple of minutes, bruise a lemongrass stalk and add into this.
5. Add the turmeric powder and stir.
6. Now add the chicken drumsticks and stir well.
7. Pour in the coconut milk and water over the chicken.
8. Sprinkle some salt and stir everything together.
9. Cover the pan and let it cook for about 15-20 minutes.
10. Once you feel the chicken is cooked, remove from heat and serve with some chopped cilantro over it.

Thai Chicken Tacos:

Ingredients:

For Marinade:

- 1/4 cup orange juice
- 2 tablespoons soy sauce
- 1 tablespoon honey
- 1/2 tablespoon ginger, grated
- 1 tablespoon lime juice
- 1/4 teaspoon red pepper flakes or to taste

For Peanut Sauce:
- 1 tablespoon peanut butter
- 1 tablespoon soy sauce
- 1 tablespoons grated ginger
- 1/2 tablespoon sesame oil
- 1 tablespoon honey
- 1/4 teaspoon red pepper flakes or to taste

For Tacos:
- 2 carrots, julienned
- 1 red pepper, deseeded, sliced thinly
- 1 medium head cabbage, remove 6 whole leaves and keep aside, thinly slice the rest of the cabbage
- 3chicken breasts
- 2 tablespoons cilantro
- 2 -3 tablespoons crushed peanuts
- Limes wedges to serve
- Sriracha sauce for serving

Method:

1. To make the marinade: Mix together all the ingredients of the marinade in a large bowl. Mix well. Add the chicken breasts. Coat well with the marinade. Cover and refrigerate overnight.
2. To make the peanut sauce: Mix together all the ingredients of the peanut sauce in a small bowl. Mix well and refrigerate.
3. Preheat a grill to medium heat. Grill the chicken pieces on both the sides for approximately 7-8 minutes per side.
4. When the grilled chicken is cool enough to handle, slice the chicken into thin slices.
5. To make the tacos: Spread the whole cabbage leaves on your working area.
6. Divide the chicken slices amongst the cabbage leaves. Place a few red pepper slices over the chicken.
7. Place some shredded cabbage and peanut sauce over the red pepper slices.
8. Sprinkle cilantro and crushed peanuts.
9. Fold over the cabbage leaves. Serve with Sriracha sauce.

Chicken Guadalajara:

Ingredients:

- 5-6 tablespoons butter
- 1 cup white onions, chopped fine
- 6 cloves garlic, minced
- 8 chicken breast halves, boneless, skinless, rinsed, pat dried, slice across into 1/2 inch thick slices
- 2 cans (12 ounces each) diced tomatoes and green chilies
- 8 ounces full fat cream cheese, cut into slices or cubes
- 1/2 cup whipping cream
- 1/2 cup chicken broth + more if required
- 1 teaspoon cayenne pepper or to taste
- 2 teaspoons dried cumin
- 1 teaspoon garlic powder or to taste
- 2 teaspoon sea salt or to taste
- Grated cheddar cheese for garnish
- Sour cream for garnish
- Salsa to serve

Method:

1. Place a large skillet over medium heat. Add butter. When the butter melts, add onions and sauté for 3-4 minutes. Add garlic and sauté until the onions are translucent.
2. Add chicken breasts and cook on all the sides until slightly brown
3. Lower the heat and add tomatoes and chilies. Cover and simmer until the chicken is cooked.

4. Add cream cheese and cream Mix well until the cheese melts and coast the chicken and the vegetables. Add more broth if the gravy is too thick.
5. Garnish with sour cream. Serve with salsa.

Chicken and peppers

Ingredients:

- 1 lb. chicken mince
- 2 Cups parmesan shredded cheese
- 3 large bell peppers, one of each color
- 2 tablespoons olive oil
- 1 red onion, chopped
- 2 tablespoons mustard
- 2 tablespoons hot sauce
- Salt to taste
- Pepper to taste

Method

1. Preheat the oven to 325 Fahrenheit
2. Place a pan on heat and add in the oil and onions and sauté until golden.
3. Add in the ground chicken and sauté until the meat is golden.
4. Add in the seasonings, mustard and hot sauce and cook on low.
5. Meanwhile, prepare the peppers by removing their cores and seeds and clean them.
6. Switch off the heat and stuff each pepper with the chicken mix.

7. Place the peppers on a baking tray sprayed with cooking spray and place in the hot oven for 45 minutes or until they are almost cooked.
8. Remove them and sprinkle the cheese on top and place it back for 15 minutes.
9. Serve hot.

Chicken Paprika:

Ingredients:

- 6 chicken breasts, skinless, boneless, chop into chunks
- 4 tablespoons olive oil
- 4 tablespoons Spanish smoked paprika
- 3 tablespoons lemon juice
- 1 1/2 tablespoons maple syrup
- 3 teaspoons garlic, minced
- Salt to taste
- Pepper powder to taste

Method:

1. Mix together all the ingredients except the chicken to make the sauce.
2. Season the chicken with salt and pepper.
3. Pour 1/3 of the sauce to a casserole dish. Place the chicken pieces on top of it.
4. Pour the remaining sauce all over the chicken pieces.
5. Bake in a preheated oven at 350 degree F for about 30 minutes or until done.
6. Broil the chicken for 4-5 minutes and serve.

Brian Adams

Chapter 20: Beef Recipes

<u>Easy Meatloaf</u>

Ingredients

- ½ cup almond flour
- ½ cup dry grated cheddar cheese
- 2 tablespoons almond butter
- 2 white onions, chopped
- 5 garlic pieces, minced
- 1 cup green pepper, sliced
- 2 large eggs
- 1 tablespoon fresh basil leaves, chopped
- 1 tablespoon thyme leaves, chopped
- ¼ cup fresh parsley leaves, chopped
- 2 tablespoons oregano leaves, chopped
- Salt to taste
- Pepper to taste

- 2 teaspoons mustard
- ¼ cup full fat cream
- ½ teaspoon unflavored gelatin
- 2 lb. ground beef, minced
- 1 pound chicken sausage

Method

1. Preheat the oven to 350 Fahrenheit.
2. Grease a large baking dish with the butter.
3. In a medium deep bowl, mix the almond flour and the cheddar cheese together and set it aside.
4. Heat the butter in a small skillet over medium heat and add in the onion, the garlic and the pepper and sauté it until golden brown.
5. Allow it to cool completely.
6. Once cool, place the mix and all the herbs in a blender and create a smooth mix.
7. In a large bowl, mix the eggs along with the spices, the salt, the pepper, the mustard and the cream and give it a good mix.
8. Add in the onion mix and mix until well combined.
9. Sprinkle the gelatin over it and set it aside.
10. Meanwhile, place the ground beef and the chicken sausage on work board and knead them until both combine and there are no big sausage pieces.
11. Add the meat mix to the egg mix and mix it until well combined and the eggs completely coat the meat.
12. Add in the almond flour and cheese mixture and mix it until well combined and grease your hands if you think it will all be a bit too sticky.

13. Place it in the baking dish covered in butter and use the back of your hands to flatten it and punch it down using your knuckles.
14. Bake it until brown or until a skewer inserted in the center comes out clean.
15. This can take anywhere from 1 hour to 1 and a half hours.
16. Serve hot.

Ground Beef and Spinach Skillet:

Ingredients:

- 4 tablespoons coconut oil or ghee
- 2 king oyster mushrooms, chopped
- 4 tablespoons raw almonds, chopped
- 300 grams grass fed ground beef
- ½ teaspoon chili pepper flakes
- A large pinch Himalayan salt
- A large pinch ground white pepper
- ½ cup pitted kalamata olives
- 2 tablespoons capers
- 2 tablespoons natural roasted almond butter
- 300 grams baby spinach leaves, roughly chopped

Method:

1. Place a heavy bottomed skillet over medium high heat. Add coconut oil. When oil is melted, add mushrooms and sauté until brown.
2. Almonds and sauté for a minute. Add beef, salt, white pepper powder, chili pepper flakes and cook until the meat is brown and cooked well.
3. Add olives, capers and almond butter. Mix well. Add spinach and sauté for a couple of minutes until the spinach wilts well.
4. Serve immediately.

Crispy Sesame Beef:

Ingredients:

- 2 medium daikon radish (about 1.5 pound)
- 2 pounds rib-eye steak, sliced into ¼" strips
- 2 tablespoons coconut flour
- 1 teaspoon guar gum
- 2 tablespoons coconut oil
- ½ cup soy sauce
- 2 teaspoons sesame oil
- 2 teaspoons oyster sauce
- 3 tablespoons rice vinegar
- 2 teaspoons Sriracha
- 1 teaspoon red pepper flakes
- 2 tablespoons sesame seeds, toasted
- 1 medium red pepper, sliced into thin strips
- 1 medium jalapeno pepper, thinly sliced
- 2 medium green onion, chopped
- 2 cloves garlic, minced
- 2 teaspoons ginger, minced
- 10 drops Liquid Stevia (optional)
- Oil for frying

Method:

1. Using a spiralizer, make noodles of the daikon radish. Alternately, using a julienne peeler, make noodles of the radish.

2. Soak the noodles in cold water about 20-25 minutes. Drain and keep aside.
3. Place a large frying pan or wok over high heat. When the oil is heated, add ginger, garlic and red pepper. Sauté for a couple of minutes until fragrant. Add sesame seeds and sauté for a couple of minutes.
4. Add soy sauce, oyster sauce, sesame oil, vinegar, Sriracha and stevia. Mix well and let it cook for a couple of minutes. Remove from heat.
5. Meanwhile, place a deep pan over medium heat. Pour oil in it such that it covers at least an inch in height from the bottom of the pan.
6. When the oil is hot enough for frying (temperature of the oil should be nearly 325 degree F) add beef strips in batches and cook on both the sides until brown and crisp.
7. Remove the strips by a slotted spoon. Place on paper towels.
8. Reheat the wok. Add the crispy beef strips and sauté for a couple of minutes.
9. To serve: Place some daikon noodles on a serving plate. Top with a few crispy beef strips and serve.

Reuben Casserole:

Ingredients:

- 3/4 pound corned beef, diced
- 3/4 can sauerkraut, drained
- 1 1/2 cups Swiss cheese, shredded
- 6 tablespoons mayonnaise
- 6 ounces cream cheese
- 6 tablespoons low sugar ketchup
- 2 tablespoons pickle brine or ½ teaspoon vinegar,
- 1/2 teaspoon caraway seeds

Method:

1. Heat a saucepan over low heat. Add cream cheese, mayonnaise, and ketchup. When melted add half the Swiss cheese, sauerkraut and beef. Mix until well combined and cheese is melted.
2. Remove from heat and add pickle brine. Mix well. Transfer into a greased baking dish.
3. Sprinkle with the remaining cheese and caraway seeds.
4. Bake in a preheated oven at 350 degrees F for until the cheese is slightly browned.
5. Serve hot.

Brian Adams

Chapter 21: Pork Recipes

<u>Ground Pork Tacos:</u>

Ingredients:

- 2 pounds ground pork
- 1 1/2 teaspoons garlic powder
- 1 1/2 teaspoons onion powder
- 1 1/2 teaspoon sea salt
- 1 teaspoon ground cumin
- 1/2 teaspoon ground pepper or to taste
- 1/4 cup salsa
- 15 large lettuce leaves or more if required
- 3/4 cup green bell pepper, chopped
- 3/4 cup red bell pepper, chopped
- 2 medium onions, chopped

Brian Adams

Method:

1. Add pork to a frying pan. Add garlic powder, onion powder, salt, cumin, and pepper. Mix well using your hands.
2. Place the pan over medium heat. Stir constantly and cook until the pork is browned well
3. Remove the pork with a slotted spoon and place in a bowl. Discard the remaining fat.
4. Add salsa and mix well. Taste and adjust the seasonings if necessary
5. Lay the lettuce leaves on your working area. Place some pork filling at the center.
6. Sprinkle peppers, and onions. Roll and serve.

Italian pork cutlets:

Ingredients:

- 15 pork cutlets
- 1 1/2 cups Italian salsa
- 1/2 cup parmesan cheese, grated
- 2 tablespoons Italian seasoning or to taste

Method:

1. Place the Italian dressing in a bowl. Add seasonings.

2. Place the cheese in another bowl.

3. Place a frying pan on medium heat. Dip the cutlets in the Italian dressing.

4. Next roll it in the cheese, and place in it the pan. Cook on both the sides until brown and cooked through.

5. Serve hot with Italian salsa.

Brian Adams

Bacon Wrapped Pork Tenderloin:

Ingredients:

- 1 tenderloin (2 pounds), pat dried
- 5 slices bacon
- 1 tablespoon Dijon mustard
- 1 tablespoon sugar free maple syrup
- 1/2 tablespoon soy sauce
- 1 teaspoon garlic, minced
- 1/2 teaspoon liquid smoke
- 1/2 teaspoon dried rosemary
- Black pepper powder to taste
- 1/4 teaspoon cayenne pepper
- 1/4 teaspoon dried sage

Method:

1. Mix together all the ingredients except pork and bacon in a large bowl. Add pork to it. Mix well and transfer the entire contents of the bowl to a zip lock bag. Shake well and refrigerate for at least 4 - 5 hours.
2. Remove from the refrigerator and place on a foiled baking sheet. Wrap the tenderloin with the bacon slices.
3. Bake in a preheated oven for about an hour.
4. Broil for 5-7 minutes. Remove from oven and cover loosely for 8-10 minutes.
5. Cut into pieces and serve.

Chapter 22: Seafood Recipes

Baked Salmon:

Ingredients:

- 6 salmon fillets (around 6 ounces each)
- 6 cloves garlic, minced
- 12 tablespoons light olive oil
- 3 teaspoons dried basil
- 1 1/2 teaspoons salt or to taste
- 1 teaspoon freshly ground black pepper or to taste
- 3 tablespoons lemon juice
- 3 tablespoons fresh parsley, chopped

Method:

1. Add to a glass dish, garlic, oil, basil, salt, pepper, lemon juice and parsley. Whisk well.

2. Add salmon and stir well. Place in the refrigerator for marinating for at least an hour. Turn the salmon a couple of times in between.
3. Transfer the salmon along with marinade in aluminum foil. Seal well.
4. Bake it in an ovenproof dish for about 45 minutes in a preheated oven at 375 degree F.

Sri Lankan Fish Curry

Ingredients:

- 6 pieces (200grams each) Silver Hake or any other white fish
- 6 tablespoons coconut oil
- ½ teaspoon whole mustard seeds
- 3 long green chilies, deseeded, cut in small pieces
- 1/2-tablespoon fresh ginger, grated.
- 1/2 teaspoon ground cumin
- 1/2 tablespoon curry powder
- 2 inch fresh turmeric root, grated or 3/4 teaspoon ground turmeric powder
- 1 red onion, finely chopped
- 5 cloves of garlic, chopped
- 2 1/2 cups full fat coconut cream
- 1 teaspoon sea salt
- Chopped cilantro to garnish
- 3/4 cup water

Method:

1. Place a large saucepan over medium heat. Add half the coconut oil. When the oil is melted, add mustard seeds. In a while, it will start spluttering. When the sound of spluttering reduces, add onions and sauté for a few minutes.
2. Add ginger and garlic. Sauté for 4-5 minutes.
3. Add green chilies, curry powder, cumin powder and turmeric. Sauté for a couple of minutes more.
4. Add coconut milk and salt. Mix well and bring to a boil.

5. Reduce heat and simmer for about 15 minutes.
6. Meanwhile, add rest of the oil to a nonstick pan. Place the pan over medium heat.
7. Add fish to it and fry for 2 -3 minutes. Flip sides in between.
8. Add fish to the simmering curry. Simmer for another 5-7 minutes.
9. Serve garnished with cilantro.

Shrimp and Bacon skillet:

Ingredients:

- 8 slices uncured bacon, cut into 1 inch pieces
- 2 cups mushrooms, sliced
- 8 ounces smoked salmon, cut into strips
- 8 ounces raw shelled shrimp
- 1 cup heavy whipping cream
- A large pinch Celtic sea salt
- Freshly ground black pepper to taste

Method:

1. Place a large cast iron skillet over medium heat. Add bacon. Cook until done.
2. Add mushrooms and sauté until tender.
3. Add smoked salmon. Sauté for 2-3 minutes.
4. Add cream and salt. Reduce heat and simmer for a minute.
5. Serve immediately with zucchini noodles.

Brian Adams

Chapter 23: Lamb Recipes

Pan grilled Lamb Chops and Cardoons

Ingredients:

- 3 lamb shoulder chops
- 3 cloves garlic
- 2 sprigs fresh rosemary
- 5 tablespoons olive oil
- Celtic sea salt to taste

For cardoons:

- 2 bunch cardoons, peel the outer hard skin, cut into 4 inch long pieces
- Celtic sea salt to taste

Method:

1. To make the lamb chops: Blend together garlic, rosemary, salt and oil in a blender until well combined
2. Place the lamb chops in a bowl. Rub the chops with the oil mixture. Cover and keep aside for about 1/2 an hour.
3. Place a cast iron skillet over medium heat. When the skillet is nice and hot (when a few drops of water is sprinkled, it should sizzle), add lamb chops and grill on both the sides until done. Remove the lamb pieces and keep aside. Let the juices remain in the skillet.
4. To make the cardoons: Place a large saucepan with about a liter of water to boil. Add salt. Add cardoons and cook until tender. Drain and keep aside.
5. Reheat the skillet. Add the cooked cardoons. Heat thoroughly.
6. Serve the lamb chops topped with cardoons.

Lamb Souvlaki (Greek Lamb Skewers):

Ingredients:

- 2 1/2 pounds lamb, chopped into medium size pieces
- 1/2 cup fresh mint, chopped or 2 teaspoons dried mint
- 3 tablespoons fresh rosemary, chopped or 2 teaspoons dried rosemary
- Juice of 2 lemons
- 3/4 cup extra virgin olive oil
- 1 teaspoon salt or to taste
- Melitzanosalata to serve

Method:

1. Add olive oil and lemon juice to a large bowl. Add salt, mint, and rosemary to it and mix well.
2. Add the lamb pieces and mix well. Marinate in the refrigerator overnight. Toss it a couple of times in between.
3. Thread the meat pieces on to skewers. Place the skewers on the rack in a preheated oven.
4. Roast at 450 degree F until done. Turn the skewers around a couple of times.
5. Remove from the oven. Let it cool for a couple of minutes. Remove from the skewers.
6. Serve with Melitzanosalata.

Chapter 24: Smoothie Recipes

<u>Green Smoothie:</u>

Ingredients:

- 1 ½ cup coconut milk, unsweetened
- 3 cups baby spinach, rinsed, drained
- 1 banana, peeled, sliced
- 3 tablespoons almond butter
- 2 teaspoons vanilla extract
- 2 scoops protein powder
- Few cubes of ice
- 2 -3 tablespoons chia seeds

Method:

1. Add all the ingredients to a blender and blend until smooth.
2. Serve immediately.

Brian Adams

Chocolate Smoothie:

Ingredients:

- 2 cups, almond milk, unsweetened
- Few drops stevia or honey or agave nectar any other artificial sweetener to taste
- 1/2 cup heavy cream
- 3 scoops chocolate flavored whey powder
- Ice cubes as required
- Crushed ice to serve (optional)

Method:

1. Place all the ingredients in a blender and blend until smooth.
2. Pour into tall glasses.
3. Serve immediately with crushed ice.

Fat Bomb Smoothie Recipe:

Ingredients:

- 3 cups coconut milk
- 3 cups heavy cream
- ¼ cup unrefined coconut oil
- 3 cups strawberries
- A pinch of salt
- Few cubes ice

Method:

1. Place all the ingredients in a blender and blend until smooth.
2. Pour into tall glasses.
3. Serve immediately with crushed ice.

Peanut Butter – Banana Smoothie:

Ingredients:

- 1 cup skim milk
- 1 cup fat free plain yogurt
- ¼ cup creamy peanut butter, unsalted
- ½ ripe banana (an over ripe banana will do the best), peeled, chopped
- 2 tablespoons honey
- Ice cubes

Method:

1. Place all the ingredients in a blender and blend until smooth.
2. Pour into tall glasses.
3. Serve immediately with crushed ice.

Green Goddess Smoothie:

Ingredients:

- 2 cups water
- 1 ½ head romaine lettuce, chopped
- 5 stalks celery, trimmed, chopped
- 1 large apple, cored, chopped
- 1 pear, cored, chopped
- 1 large ripe banana, peeled, chopped
- 2-3 teaspoons lemon juice
- 1/2 cup parsley, chopped
- 1/2 cup cilantro, chopped
- A handful of mint leaves (optional)
- 1/2 cup spinach
- Ice as required

Method:

1. Place all the ingredients in a blender and blend until smooth.
2. Pour into tall glasses.
3. Serve immediately with crushed ice.

Perfect Vegan Smoothie:

Ingredients:

- 1 cup frozen strawberries
- 1 cup frozen raspberries
- 1 cup frozen blueberries
- 1 cup frozen blackberries
- 2 cups kale, stems, tough ribs removed, roughly chopped
- 2 cups spinach
- 2 cups ripe bananas, peeled, chopped
- 1 cup orange juice
- 1 cup pomegranate juice
- 1/2 cup soft tofu
- Ice cubes as required

Method:

1. Place all the ingredients in a blender and blend until smooth.
2. Pour into tall glasses.
3. Serve immediately with crushed ice.

Healthy Breakfast Smoothie:

Ingredients:

- 3 cups frozen raspberries
- 2 cups almond milk, unsweetened
- 1 cup frozen cherries, pitted
- 3 tablespoons honey or to taste
- 2 tablespoons fresh ginger, peeled, grated
- 2 teaspoons ground flaxseeds
- 1 tablespoon lemon juice
- Ice cubes as required

Method:

1. Place all the ingredients in a blender and blend until smooth.
2. Pour into tall glasses.
3. Serve immediately with crushed ice.

Brian Adams

Chapter 25: Desserts Recipes

Choco-chip muffins

Ingredients:

- 1 cup of almond flour
- ½ cup of cream
- 1 egg
- 4 tbsp of butter
- 4 tbsp of xylitol
- 1 tsp of baking soda
- 1 tsp of vanilla extract
- Sprinkle of salt
- Handful of chocolate chips

Method:

1. Preheat the oven to 370 degrees.

2. In a bowl, mix the cream into the almond flour. Add the egg into this and stir well.
3. Then add melted butter with the baking soda, xylitol, salt and vanilla extract.
4. Mix everything well and add the chocolate chips. Stir well to distribute evenly.
5. Scoop out the mixture into cupcake molds and bake for 15 minutes.
6. Serve after cooling.

No bake Cheesecake

Ingredients:

- 100 gms of cream cheese
- 50 gms heavy cream
- ½ tsp of Glycerite
- 1 tsp of powdered sweetener (low carb)
- 1 tbsp of lemon juice
- 1 tsp of vanilla essence

Method:

1. Mix all the ingredients together in a bowl.
2. Whip them into a pudding like consistency.
3. Then scoop into cups and let it set in the fridge.
4. Serve.

<u>Chocolate pudding</u>

Ingredients:

- 200 gm of cream cheese
- 100 gm of whipping cream
- 4 drops of liquid stevia
- 30 gm of grated dark chocolate (90 % cocoa)

Method:

1. Take a bowl and just mix all the ingredients together. Mash it all up well.
2. Scoop into bowls and let it sit in the fridge till they set.

Chocolate brownies for Dessert

Ingredients

- 2 cups Almond Flour
- 1/2 cup Cocoa Powder, unsweetened
- 1/3 cup Erythritol
- 1/4 cup Coconut Oil or MCT oil
- 1/4 cup Maple Syrup, low sugar
- 2 large eggs
- 1 tablespoon psyllium husk powder
- 2 tablespoons salted caramel
- 1 teaspoon baking Powder
- 1/2 teaspoon salt

Method

1. Preheat the oven to 350 Fahrenheit.
2. Place the oil, maple syrup, eggs and caramel in a bowl and whisk until well combined.
3. Place the flour, cocoa powder, sugar, husk, baking powder and salt in a sieve and sieve it to get rid of impurities.
4. Add the dry mix to the wet and use a blender to whisk until well combined.
5. Place the mix in a greased brownie tray and place it in the oven for 20 minutes or until a skewer inserted in the center comes out clean.
6. Allow it to cool on a wire rack for 30 minutes to an hour, slice it and serve it.

Chia Pudding

Ingredients:

- 4 tbsp of chia seeds
- 1 cup of Almond milk
- A handful of strawberries

Method:

1. Add the chia seeds to the almond milk and let it sit in the fridge for a while.
2. While serving, slice up the strawberries and add to your pudding.

Strawberry smoothie

Ingredients:

- 1 ½ cup of unsweetened almond milk
- 1/3 cup of strawberries
- 1 tbsp of whey protein powder
- 2 tbsp of cream

Method:

1. Pour the almond milk into a blender.
2. Cut up the strawberries and add along with the heavy cream and protein powder.
3. Run the blender till you get the desired consistency.

Cinnamon Churritos:

Ingredients:

- 3 cups almond flour
- 1/3 cup coconut flour
- 3/4 teaspoon baking powder
- 6 teaspoons ground cinnamon, divided
- 1/2 teaspoon salt
- 3/4 cup coconut milk
- 3 tablespoons unsalted butter
- 6 tablespoons granular sugar substitute like xylitol, divided
- 3 large eggs
- Oil for deep frying

Method:

1. Place oil for deep-frying in a shallow skillet or a deep fryer. Oil should cover at least 2-3 inches height from the bottom of the skillet. Heat oil to 375 degree F.
2. Meanwhile make the dry mixture as follows: Mix together almond flour, coconut flour, baking powder, half the cinnamon and salt. Keep aside
3. Place a saucepan over medium heat. Pour the coconut milk. Add butter, and 3 tablespoons xylitol. Bring to a boil.
4. Remove from heat. Add the dry mixture to this and mix well until it is thick and resembles a dough.
5. Let it cool for 10 minutes.

6. Add the eggs and mix again to form a thick paste.
7. Drop tablespoons of this mixture into the hot oil. About 5-6 per batch. Fry until golden brown.
8. Turn the Churritos on all sides so that it is evenly brown.
9. Remove with a slotted spoon and place on paper towels until the next batch is ready.
10. Repeat step 7 - 9 with the remaining batter.
11. Pulse together the xylitol and cinnamon in a blender to make the xylitol granules slightly finer. Transfer on to a plate.
12. Roll the fried Churritos over the xylitol – cinnamon mixture. Coat well.
13. Serve immediately if you like it hot or serve it at room temperature

Brian Adams

Berry Ice cream:

Ingredients:

- 3 cups heavy whipping cream
- 1 1/2 cups blueberries or strawberries, unsweetened
- Few drops of stevia sweetener or any other sweetener of your choice (optional)

Method:

1. Add all the ingredients to a blender. Blend   until smooth.
2. Freeze the ice cream for 5-6 hours or until set.
3. Remove from the freezer around 30 minutes before serving.
4. Garnish with the berries that you are using.

Creamy Peanut Butter Dessert:

Ingredients:

- 6 tablespoons peanut butter, unsalted
- Sweetener of your choice
- 1/2 cup whipped cream
- 1 tablespoon cocoa powder

Method:

1. Divide the peanut butter and place in 4 individual bowls (about 1 1/2 tablespoons)
2. Sprinkle sweetener over it.
3. Spread some cream over the peanut butter.
4. Sprinkle cocoa powder over the cream.
5. Divide the remaining cream (if it is remaining) amongst the bowls and serve.

Chocolate Cake in a mug:

Ingredients:

- Cooking spray
- 3 eggs, well beaten
- 6tablespoons cocoa powder
- 6 tablespoons sugar substitute of your choice or to taste
- A pinch salt
- 3 tablespoons heavy cream
- 1 1/2 teaspoon vanilla extract
- 3/4 teaspoon baking powder
- Whipped cream to serve
- Berries of your choice to serve

Method:

1. Place together all the dry ingredients in a bowl and mix well.
2. Add cream, vanilla, and egg and whisk well.
3. Pour the batter into mugs greased with cooking spray. (½ fill it)
4. Microwave on high for about 60-80 seconds or until the top of the cake is slightly hardened.
5. Cool and invert on to individual plates. Serve with whipped cream and berries.

Blueberry Mousse:

Ingredients:

- 3 cups blueberries
- 3 cups firm tofu, drained, crumbled
- 5 tablespoons agave sweetener
- Dark dairy-free chocolate, shaved to serve

Method:

1. Add blueberries to the blender and blend.
2. Add tofu and blend until smooth. Add agave syrup and blend until well combined.
3. Transfer into individual serving bowls. Refrigerate for 3-4 hours before serving.
4. Serve garnished with chocolate shavings and a few blueberries.

Strawberry Cheese Cake:

Ingredients:

- 1 cup cream cheese, softened
- 1/2 cup heavy cream
- 4 eggs
- 2 teaspoons lemon juice
- 1 teaspoon vanilla extract
- Sugar substitute like stevia to taste
- 1 cup frozen strawberries, thawed
- Whipped cream to serve

Method:

1. Place all the ingredients in a microwave safe bowl. Whisk well until smooth.
2. Microwave on high for 90 seconds stirring in between.
3. Cool and refrigerate.
4. Serve chilled with fresh strawberry slices and whipped cream or any low carb sauce

Conclusion

The low carb or ketogenic diet can have a lasting impact on your body, as long as you do it the right way. You need to follow the basics of the diet if you want to see positive results coming through.

The thing to remember is low carb diets are not just about the carbs – everything you eat plays a part in the success of the diet, so you need to understand the basic principles of the diet, and realize why you're doing the things you do. Everything happens for a reason, and you need to be up to speed on all that.

If you think you will be able to see results within a week or two of starting on the diet, then you need to think again, frankly. The body needs to adjust to the demands of the diet and you must allow it sufficient time to do what it needs to do. This time frame depends on your body and how fast or slow your metabolism works. People have lost up to 2 pounds a day after starting out on the ketogenic diet, but as we've stressed before, everyone is different, and reacts to the diet in different ways, so there is no standard response to low carb or ketogenic dieting.

The way to succeed is to read up as much as you can about low carb dieting, so you can understand the principles underlying what you are embarking upon. It's all about the relationship between your body and the food you put into it. Low carb diets aim to force your body to burn off fat in order to achieve the figure you want and deserve. However, it isn't just a matter of cutting the carbs and waiting for the offers to roll in. You need to understand the roles played by fats and proteins in your diet too.

It is possible to adapt your lifestyle to work with low carb dieting, but because the science behind it is important too, it may be a good idea to get your physician involved with this. Nobody knows you better, and he can help you deal with any setbacks or complications along the way.

Above all, remember that low carb dieting is a long-term plan, rather than diets you 'go on' and 'come off' like a playground merry go round. If you want to burn off excess fat and feel better about yourself, you need to stick with it for at least six months, and maybe even more. You didn't get fat overnight, so you can't expect to get thin in a heartbeat, although you will see great results in both fat loss and body composition. Low carb dieting can give you the body you want and deserve, but you need to give it time to work its magic.

www.ingramcontent.com/pod-product-compliance
Lightning Source LLC
Chambersburg PA
CBHW071039290526
45795CB00004B/1217